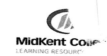

# Medical Care of the Elderly

**M R P HALL** BM BCh FRCP FRCPE
*Professor of Geriatric Medicine*
*University of Southampton*

**W J MacLENNAN** MD FRCP (Lond, Ed & Glas)
*Reader in Geriatric Medicine,*
*Department of Medicine,*
*University of Dundee*

**M D W LYE** MD FRCP
*Professor of Geriatric Medicine,*
*University of Liverpool*

## SECOND EDITION

A Wiley Medical Publication

**JOHN WILEY & SONS**
Chichester · New York · Brisbane · Toronto · Singapore

© M R P Hall, W J MacLennan, M D W Lye, 1978, 1986

*Library of Congress Cataloging-in-Publication Data:*

Hall, Michael R. P.
  Medical care of the elderly.

  (A Wiley medical publication)
  Includes bibliographies and index.
  1. Geriatrics.   2. Aged—Care and hygiene.
I. MacLennan, W. J.   II. Lye, M. D. W.   III. Title.
IV. Series.   [DNLM: 1. Aged.   2. Geriatrics.   3. Health
Services for the Aged—case studies.   WT 30 H178m]
RC952.H245   1986        362.1'9897        85-22692
ISBN 0 471 90906 8 (pbk.)

*British Library Cataloguing in Publication Data:*

Hall, M. R. P.
  Medical care of the elderly.—2nd ed.
  1. Geriatrics
  1. Title   II. MacLennan, W. J.   III. Lye, M. D. W.
  618.97        RC952

  ISBN 0 471 90906 8

Typeset by Acorn Bookwork, Salisbury, Wilts.
Printed and bound in Great Britain.

# Contents

# Preface

In the seven years that have passed since publication of the first edition of this book, the numbers of elderly have, as forecast, increased, particularly in the older age groups – those over 75 and those over 85 years of age. Consequently, a greater burden has been placed on geriatric medical resources and geriatric medicine has responded to this challenge by improving bed turnover and increasing the workload of those involved in the medical care of the elderly. This heavier workload and concomitant experience has increased and advanced clinical geriatric skills and knowledge so that much more is now known about the clinical problems posed by the older elderly than ever before. As a consequence, we have made many changes in the text of this second edition and parts of it have been completely rewritten.

Yet in spite of these alterations, which have led to a slight overall expansion of the material, we have retained the main theme of our book. It is that attitudinal and cooperative skills are necessary to treat old people successfully and that the key to this lies in our ability to understand that they are not patients, clients, senior citizens, old age pensioners or geriatrics, but people like ourselves who have a life to continue to live and a rôle, often an important one, still to play in society and life. These basic tenets have not altered with the passage of time nor do we expect that they will change in the future. We have also resisted the temptation to expand the content of the chapters to include all new advances in knowledge in each field. This knowledge can be obtained from study of the larger textbooks of geriatric medicine or from some of the specialist texts which are now being published and we have referred to some of these in the 'further reading' bibliographies at the end of each chapter.

We have retained the original form of the book, although we have added two new case histories. We feel that we are justified in taking this view because the most effective approach to the elderly patient and his problems is that of the team: our book was and is intended as a guide for this team. We have attempted an integrated approach and have tried to concentrate on the need to develop it, with each member of the team playing his own specific part in patient management. For this reason, we have avoided a specific chapter on some subjects, for example, rehabilitation and pharmacology, preferring to include such topics within the framework of the chapters.

We hope we have managed to update our book without adding too greatly to its length. We feel that it has an important place as a handbook not only for those already working in the field of the care of the elderly, irrespective of their discipline, but also for those coming into the field, to help them all to achieve a better understanding of the problems of the elderly sick.

*October, 1985*

M R P Hall
W J MacLennan
M D W Lye

# Acknowledgements

We acknowledge the help and forebearance of our secretaries, Ms Maureen Hughes and Mrs Rita Ward, in preparing this book.

# Case Histories

## 1  Female, aged 80 years

**History**  This patient was referred because she was failing to manage adequately at home. Her problems were:

(i) intermittent falls (Chapter 8: *falls*),
(ii) intermittent episodes of confusion (Chapter 9: *acute brain failure*).

Shortly before her referral she had fallen and lain on the ground for some time. The general practitioner had referred her to the social services for residential care but the assessing social worker felt that she was unsuitable because of her mental confusion and suggested a geriatric medical opinion. She was seen at home and it was felt that she could be investigated on an out-patient basis. Pending investigation she was admitted temporarily for a two-week period to a residential home.

She felt that her main problem was unsteadiness which tended to cause her to fall and reduced her mobility. She attributed this to arthritis which while mainly affecting her knees, also affected her back and shoulders and had been present for many years. She had fallen on many occasions and had in the past sustained Colles' fractures of both wrists. Her falls were of three kinds.

Firstly, she would sometimes fall without any warning and then be unable to get up, having to lie on the ground for about ten minutes until she was able to pull herself together.

Secondly, she sometimes fell because she was giddy. The giddiness caused her to lose balance; it might occur at any time and had no particular association.

Lastly, she suffered from skeletal instability caused by her arthritis, which restricted her mobility and her ability to correct errors of movement and resulted in loss of balance. She also had deformed feet as a result of bunions (hallux valgus) which had been operated on in the past.

In addition she complained of pins and needles in both hands, symptoms she had had for some months, which limited her ability to do up buttons and dress herself, as well as to pick up small things from the floor. X-ray of the cervical spine showed mild spondylitic changes (Chapter 7: *axial joints*). She thought that her mental confusion had improved,

1

although she was still easily flustered and might become confused if rushed.

Additional problems included poor vision in the right eye for 6 years (Chapter 6: *vision*) which made her clumsy; she said that the blindness had resulted from a stroke. (In fact, however, this had followed thrombosis of the right inferior temporal branch of the retinal artery thereby involving the macula. She had seen an eye specialist and no treatment was possible.) Five years earlier she had a growth (fibrosarcoma) excised from the right calf and this was associated with weakness of the (right) leg. Finally, two years earlier she had been found to have diabetes mellitus (Chapter 13: *diabetes*). An electrocardiograph done at this time showed a left bundle branch block and evidence of left ventricular hypertrophy – signs often associated with a raised arterial blood pressure (Chapter 10: *hypertension*). She was receiving tolbutamide 500 mg three times daily for her diabetes and phenylbutazone 100 mg three times daily for her arthritis.

**Examination** On examination she was found to be a grey-haired lady with puffiness under the eyes and obviously unsteady on her feet, walking with a wide-based gait. Her feet were deformed by operations for hallux valgus. She had three ischaemic ulcers on the right foot which were inflamed and discharging (Chapter 10: *peripheral arteries*). No pulse could be felt in the right foot and the radial arteries were thick and tortuous. Her pulse was irregular and slow (the ECG showed sinus rhythm with multiple extrasystoles and left bundle branch block. Chapter 10: *abnormal rhythms*).

Her heart sounds were normal but she had an apical systolic murmur and a mitral diastolic murmur. Her heart was enlarged to the left and the apex beat was left ventricular in type. In spite of this her blood pressure was only 130/70. She had a sacral pad of oedema and basal crepitations but the jugular venous pressure was not elevated. She was mildly breathless on exertion and, therefore, had some of the features of heart failure.

Examination of the central nervous system showed bilateral extensor plantar responses and no ankle jerks, but otherwise normal reflexes and no inversion of the supinator reflexes. Some muscular weakness of the right lower leg was present.

Examination of the abdomen showed a loaded colon with abdominal masses which were almost certainly faecal in origin.

**Diagnosis** This patient represented an extremely complex problem from both the medical and the social points of view. For the major problem, falls, three causes seemed possible:

1 drop attacks due to: (*a*) old age, (*b*) vertebrobasilar insufficiency (Chapter 8: *falls*);

2 muscular skeletal instability due to arthritis, weakness of right leg and paraplegia (Chapter 7: *peripheral joints; axial joints*); and
3 hypoglycaemia due to drug interaction (Chapter 13: *oral hypoglycaemics*).

To confirm these she had physical signs compatible with a diagnosis of paraplegia, indicating a lesion of the spinal cord which could be linked either to cervical spondylosis or to diabetes mellitus. The pins and needles affecting her hands might be a symptom of cervical spondylosis. Her diabetes was being treated with an oral hypoglycaemic agent which interacted with the phenylbutazone which she was receiving for her arthritis. It was possible, therefore, that too low a level of blood sugar (hypoglycaemia) could contribute to her giddiness. Similarly, this condition might also be causing her intermittent mental confusion.

Her arthritis and foot deformities added to her instability and immobility. Additional medical problems related to:

1 an overloaded bowel which could be associated with the paraplegia (Chapter 14: *faecal impaction*);
2 heart murmurs which suggested a damaged heart valve (Chapter 10: *valvular heart disease*). This latter state was undoubtedly the cause for mild heart failure (Chapter 10: *congestive cardiac failure*); and
3 arteriosclerosis (perhaps linked to the diabetes) causing:
    (i) peripheral vascular disease with ischaemic ulcers of the right foot (Chapter 13: *complications of diabetes;* Chapter 10: *peripheral arteries*),
    (ii) blindness in the right eye due to retinal artery thrombosis,
    (iii) vertebrobasilar arterial insufficiency in association with cervical spondylosis (Chapter 7: *axial joints*).

**Management**   Obviously the further care of this patient at home will be difficult. Nevertheless, she is unwilling to live permanently in an old people's home though she will go there temporarily for a period of relief (Chapter 4: *residential accommodation*). Her objection to a permanent place was that the central heating makes it too hot! However, in order to plan her continuing care in the community her case will need to be discussed in detail with the general practitioner, home nursing services, health visitor and social worker (Chapter 4: *attitudes to social problems*). The remedial therapist will need to visit and assess her home to see whether simple alterations or aids will enable her to live there more safely (Chapter 5: *adjustment of the environment*). The district housing authorities may need to be consulted and the possibility of rehousing in sheltered accommodation considered (Chapter 4: *Social Problems and the Elderly*).

SUMMARY

| Medical problems (diagnosis) | Possible effects | Possible actions |
|---|---|---|
| 1 Old age 'drop attack' | (i) 'Fall'<br>(ii) Risk of: (a) fracture, (b) hypothermia | (a) Teach to get up from floor (PT)<br>(b) Alarm system in home at floor level (SW)<br>(c) Blankets within reach of floor (HV) |
| 2 Cervical spondylosis | (i) In association with 3(iii)<br>(ii) Drop attack – fall (see 1(i)) | (a) 1(a), (b) and (c)<br>(b) Cervical collar trial (PT) |
| 3 Arteriosclerosis | (i) Peripheral vascular disease with leg ulcers<br><br>(ii) Blindness in right eye<br><br>(iii) Vertebro-basilar insufficiency<br>(iv) Brain failure<br>(v) Cerebral infarction | (a) Dressing to ulcers (N)<br>(b) Vasodilator drugs? (D)<br>(c) Control of diabetes (D, N)<br>(a) ? Blind registration (D)<br>(b) Organisation of personal environment (OT)<br>See 2(a) and 1(b)<br>Test mental function (D) |
| 4 Diabetes mellitus | (i) Arteriosclerosis<br>(ii) Cataract<br>(iii) CNS lesions (vascular and others) | See 3(i)(c) and (ii)(a)<br>Keep left eye under review (D)<br>(a) Diet (D, HV, Dtn)<br>(b) Hypoglycaemic drugs (D) |
| 5 'Arthritis' | (i) Pain<br><br><br>(ii) Diminished movement<br><br><br>(iii) Muscular atrophy<br><br>(iv) Sub-nutrition | (a) Define type, extent and severity, eg. osteoarthritis or rheumatoid (D)<br>(b) Give analgesics to control pain (D)<br>(a) Local treatment to affected joints, viz. ice (acute), heat, active movements, splints (PT)<br>Ensure ability to perform activities of daily living (OT)<br>Ensure appropriate diet (HV, SW, Dtn) |

| Medical problems (diagnosis) | Possible effects | Possible actions |
|---|---|---|
| 6 Mitral valve disease | Heart failure | (a) Give diuretics and potassium supplements (D)<br>(b) ? surgical replacement of valve (D) |
| 7 Faecal impaction | (i) Diarrhoea<br>(ii) Incontinence of urine and faeces | (a) Give laxative and softening agent (D)<br>(b) Give enemas (N)<br>(c) Increase fluid intake and dietary residue (Dtn, HV)<br>(d) Increase mobility and activity (PT) |
| 8 Drug therapy | (i) Drug interaction – hypoglycaemia, e.g. tolbutamide and phenylbutazone<br>(ii) Side effects, eg. hypotension with diuretics | Prescribe as few drugs as possible and beware interactions and adverse reactions (D) |
| 9 Live alone | (i) Needs to be able to cook and shop<br>(ii) Needs to be independent for self-care<br>(iii) Will require help if unable<br>(iv) May become lonely and isolated | (a) Assessment of ability to perform acts of daily living (OT)<br>(b) Assessment of physical activities (PT)<br>(c) Provide home help, meals-on-wheels, aids (SW)<br>(d) Rehouse in sheltered housing (HM)<br>(e) Arrange social contacts, day centre, luncheon club, pensioner club, etc. (HV, SW) |

*Key:* D = *Doctor*; HV = *Health visitor*; PT = *Physiotherapist*; Dtn = *Dietician*; N = *Nurse*; OT = *Occupational therapist*; SW = *Social worker or social services department*; HM = *Housing manager.*

## 2  Male, aged 86 years

**History**  The patient was referred for assessment of his ability to continue to manage at home. His main problems were those of isolation, urinary incontinence and reduced mobility.

When the visit was made there was considerable delay before the patient appeared at the front door with a walking aid. He was a good historian, who related that he had been relatively fit until he reached his mid-70s when he became troubled by increasing pain and stiffness in his hips which had now progressed to the stage that he was only able to get around using a Zimmer walking frame. His disability had been further accentuated by failing vision, which caused him to trip over obstacles and prevented him from reading or watching television. For the previous five years he had been troubled by breathlessness and swollen ankles, which were reasonably well controlled with digoxin, a diuretic and potassium supplements.

The patient was a widower who lived alone in a large four-bedroomed house having both upstairs and downstairs lavatories. His principal source of help was his daughter who lived about two miles away; she had performed all his shopping and housework but this support became more difficult when she herself developed congestive cardiac failure. The situation became more desperate four weeks previously when the old man developed urinary incontinence. He stated that he knew when he was about to pass urine, but was unable to get to the lavatory quickly enough. The breaking point came when his daughter's husband had a coronary thrombosis, and she had to spend her time supporting him at home and could not continue to visit the old man regularly.

**Examination**  During the course of the history it became apparent that the patient was alert and highly motivated. He was able to get out of a chair on his own, but walked slowly and unsteadily with small shuffling steps, leaning heavily on his walking frame. Active and passive movements were grossly restricted in both hip joints. He could see well enough to count fingers, but could not read large newspaper print. Ophthalmoscopy revealed that both lenses were clear, but there was patchy pigmentation of both maculae (areas of the retinae concerned with central vision).

His pulse was irregular with a rate of 84/min. and his lying and standing blood pressures were 185/90. His apex beat was forceful in character, and displaced outwards from the mid-clavicular line. The first and second heart sounds were rather faint, and there was a third sound in early diastole. The lung bases were clear and there was no peripheral oedema. His abdomen was not distended and showed no abnormal masses. The rectum was empty and the prostate was normal.

**Management** The problem of urinary incontinence made home care untenable and he was admitted to hospital for investigation and rehabilitation.

Several factors were aggravating this patient's incontinence.

1 Poor mobility prevented him from getting to the lavatory quickly enough. An X-ray confirmed the presence of severe osteoarthritis in both hips (Chapter 7: *peripheral joints*). He was put on to naproxen 500 mg twice daily and given a course of physiotherapy. This consisted mainly of exercises to his quadriceps and practice in walking.

2 Visual impairment placed further restrictions on his mobility. An ophthalmologist confirmed that little could be done to improve vision (Chapter 6: *macular degeneration*), and regretted that he had not seen the patient two years earlier when photocoagulation might have arrested the degenerative process in at least one eye. The only advice he could give was to try a magnifying glass, which enabled the patient to pick out large print, but made little difference to his reading ability.

3 An ECG confirmed that he had atrial fibrillation and that there were ischaemic changes in the antero-lateral leads (Chapter 10: *abnormal rhythms*). Radiography demonstrated that his heart was enlarged but both lung fields were clear. It appeared, then, that his cardiac failure was under satisfactory control (Chapter 10: *congestive cardiac failure*). Further questioning revealed that he experienced a brisk drug-induced diuresis each morning and this added considerably to the difficulty in keeping dry. The short-acting diuretic was replaced by one which had a gentler effect spread over 24 hours (Chapter 14: *diuretics*).

4 While attempts were being made to modify these aggravating factors attention was also directed to the incontinence itself. The nursing staff kept a urine chart to time the incontinence, which led to the identification of the diuretic problem and its effective modification (Chapter 14: *incontinence*). On more detailed investigation, bacteriological examination of the urine was negative and pressure recordings of bladder function (Chapter 14: *cystometrography*) and X-ray appearances (Chapter 14: *radiology*) were both normal.

5 During his stay in hospital the incontinence settled. Despite intensive physiotherapy, however, his movements remained very slow and he had considerable difficulty in getting on and off the lavatory.

This last problem was solved by using an elevated seat (Chapter 14: *environmental changes*; Chapter 5: *adjustment of the environment*). Contact with his family revealed that both his daughter and son-in-law remained in poor health and that it was unlikely that they would be able to offer much material help to him after discharge. It was also recognised that in his own house, the distance between the lavatories and the living areas was likely to exacerbate his problem. He eventually decided to move into a rest home (Chapter 4: *residential accommodation*). His daughter, told of his needs, visited several rest homes in the area and eventually selected one. An occupational therapist then visited and ensured that his bedroom was within easy reach of the main living areas and that all were near a lavatory. The patient was then discharged but was given an appointment to attend an out-patient clinic three weeks' later to ensure that no problems had been overlooked.

SUMMARY

| Medical problems (diagnosis) | Possible effects | Possible actions |
|---|---|---|
| 1 Osteoarthritis of hips | (i) Pain in hips | (a) Analgesics (D) |
| | (ii) Limited mobility | (b) Walking exercises (PT) |
| | (iii) Aggravation of incontinence | |
| | (iv) Difficulty in using lavatory | (c) Elevated lavatory seat (OT) |
| 2 Macular degeneration | (i) Visual impairment | (a) Photocoagulation (if early enough) (Sp) |
| | (ii) Limited mobility | |
| | (iii) Difficulty in reading or watching TV | (b) Talking books, large-print books, etc. (OT) |
| 3 Ischaemic heart disease | (i) Atrial fibrillation | (a) Digoxin (D) |
| | (ii) Cardiac failure | (b) Diuretic (D) |
| 4 Diuretic therapy | (i) Electrolyte imbalance | (a) Check electrolytes (D) |
| | (ii) Accentuation of incontinence | (b) Give potassium supplements (D) |
| | | (c) Change to longer-acting diuretic (D) |
| 5 Urinary incontinence | (i) Psychological distress | (a) Incontinence chart (N) |
| | (ii) Load on attendants | (b) Toilet training (N) |
| | (iii) Long-term hospital care | (c) Investigation of bladder function (pressures, radiology) (D) |
| | | (d) Management of problems 1, 2, 3 and 4 |
| 6 Isolation | (i) Loneliness | (a) Visitor (V) |
| | (ii) Malnutrition | (b) Meals-on-wheels (SW) |

| Medical problems (diagnosis) | Possible effects | Possible actions |
|---|---|---|
| | (iii) Domestic squalor | (c) Home help (SW) |
| | (iv) Lack of support in self-care | (d) Nursing aid (CN) |
| 7 Unsuitable housing | (i) Accentuation of incontinence | (a) Modification of house (SW, OT) |
| | (ii) Domestic squalor | (b) Sheltered housing (SW, HM, OT) |
| | (iii) Untidy house | (c) Rest home (SW, OT, Pr) |
| | (iv) Lack of support in self-care | |

*Key:* D = *Doctor;* N = *Nurse;* CN = *Community nurse;* OT = *Occupational therapist;*
V = *Visitor;* PT = *Physiotherapist;* SW = *Social worker;* Pr = *Proprietor of rest home;*
Sp = *Specialist;* HM = *Housing manager.*

## 3  Male, aged 65 years

**History**  This man was referred as his wife reported that he had become increasingly confused and aggressive over the previous twenty-four hours and that 'something had to be done'. When visited at home it emerged that the patient, an ex-regimental sergeant major, had been an extremely active man until his left side had become paralysed as a result of a 'stroke' eight years earlier. Though this never completely resolved he made a reasonable functional recovery only to suffer an even more severe right-sided paralysis two years later. He made very slow progress but eventually was able to get around his house with the aid of a tripod walking stick.

The situation remained reasonably satisfactory until about three months before the crisis. The wife had then noted that her husband was becoming increasingly muddled. He often could not remember whether or not he had had a meal, he mistook night for day and mis-identified relatives. Any attempt to correct him led to outbursts of aggression. Helping him to wash or dress often initiated particularly violent behaviour, which had culminated in his striking his wife on several occasions. Yet a further cause of distress was severe urinary and faecal incontinence.

**Examination**  Detailed assessment was difficult because of his restlessness. There was obvious weakness and spasticity in his right arm and leg. Neurological abnormalities were less obvious on the left side, but both plantar reflexes were extensor. Examination showed the heart and lungs to be normal, but striking features were pale conjunctivae and a red and smooth tongue. Palpation of the abdomen revealed a tender mass in the left iliac fossa, rectal examination showing the rectum loaded with hard craggy faeces.

**Management**   The first measure, on admission to hospital, was to control restlessness and aggression (Chapter 9: *acute brain failure*). An intramuscular injection of 50 mg of chlorpromazine was given, with an oral dose of 25 mg thrice daily. Attention was also directed to his faecal impaction (Chapter 14: *faecal impaction*), which was cleared by a phosphate enema followed by lactulose in a dose of 15 ml three times a day. Several enemas were required, but eventually a regular bowel movement pattern was re-established.

Attention could now be directed to the cause of his confusion (Chapter 9: *acute brain failure*). There was little doubt that he suffered from severe cerebro-vascular disease, and it was possible that this deterioration had been due to a further stroke, but there was no obvious other precipitating factor. Both carotid arteries were patent, the blood pressure was normal and the ECG showed only minor ischaemic changes (Chapter 8: *stroke illness*).

Possible causes for his mental impairment were investigated. A significant finding was that the haemoglobin was low (8.6 g/100 ml) and that individual red cells were small (microcytic) and contained little haemoglobin (hypochromic) (Chapter 12: *anaemia*; Chapter 3: *haematological tests*). A low serum—iron concentration was found, but blood folic acid and $B_{12}$ were normal. Nursing staff tested three specimens of faeces and found that all contained high concentrations of blood. The diagnosis of iron-deficiency anaemia due to blood loss was made and endoscopy by a gastro-enterologist arranged. This revealed an ulcer with heaped-up edges close to the pyloric sphincter. A biopsy contained tissue which was highly suggestive of malignancy (Chapter 12: *peptic ulcer; gastric cancer*).

There was considerable debate as to whether surgery was justified in this particular patient. It was felt, however, that anaemia and possible humoral changes produced by the tumour might be accentuating his confusion. Even if his survival was limited the quality of his life would be improved by increasing his intellectual capacity.

He was prepared for surgery by giving him a blood transfusion of four pints of packed cells over 48 hours. A partial gastrectomy was then performed and during the course of the operation he received a further two pints of blood. Despite his cerebro-vascular disease he made an uneventful post-operative recovery. His aggression settled, he became much more co-operative and formal testing revealed considerable improvement in mental function. The surgeon agreed that the ulcer looked malignant but microscopic examination showed no evidence of malignant change, only of chronic inflammation.

With correction of the alimentary lesion and control of his confusion, attention was directed to controlling his incontinence and increasing his mobility. Cystometography confirmed that he had a hypersensitive hypertonic bladder (Chapter 14: *cystometography*). He was treated with propantheline, a bladder relaxant, and put on to a two-hourly toileting *régime* (Chapter 14: *toilet training, drugs*); the incontinence settled over the course of the following week. Initially he required the support of a physiotherapist and her assistant when walking, but was soon able to walk with a frame. Parallel with this he received instruction in washing, dressing and toileting and was soon self-sufficient (Chapter 8: *management of stroke illness*).

His wife was told that he would be fit for discharge home in the near future. On hearing this she became extremely upset, for she had found his recent behaviour intolerable and was apprehensive about it recurring (Chapter 4: *attitudes in relation to social problems*; Chapter 2: *social acceptability*). It also emerged that ever since the first stroke eight years previously his personality had changed and he had become extremely demanding. As a result there had been a deterioration in their relationship and indeed, at one point, she had threatened to seek a divorce. A meeting between the patient, his wife, the medical social worker, the occupational therapist, the physiotherapists, the ward sister and the consultant was arranged (Chapter 5: *case conference*) from which a clearer picture of the domestic situation and the improvement in the patient's capacity emerged. Following this he was discharged home, with follow-up appointments at an out-patient clinic made so that his progress and behaviour at home could be supervised.

*(summary overleaf)*

SUMMARY

| Medical problems (diagnosis) | Possible effects | Possible actions |
|---|---|---|
| 1 Multiple strokes | (i) Mental impairment<br>(ii) Physical impairment | (a) Investigated for remediable causes (D)<br>(b) Arrange rehabilitation programme (PT, OT, N) |
| 2 Aggression and agitation | (i) Breakdown of support at home<br>(ii) Institutionalisation | (a) Control of initial problem with tranquillisers (D)<br>(b) Treatment of exacerbating factors, e.g. faecal impaction (D, N)<br>(c) Investigation for underlying cause (D) |
| 3 Anaemia | (i) Confusion | (a) Identify cause (D)<br>(b) Treat with transfusion (D)<br>(c) Treat with oral iron (D) |
| 4 Gastric cancer | (i) Anaemia<br>(ii) Confusion | (a) Perform radical surgery (S)<br>(b) Perform local excision (S)<br>(c) Leave alone |
| 5 Urinary incontinence | (i) Barrier to discharge<br>(ii) Source of embarrassment | (a) Control exacerbating factors, eg. faecal impaction (D, N)<br>(b) Investigate bladder function (D)<br>(c) Treat irritable bladder with anti-cholinergic agent (D)<br>(d) Arrange programme of toilet training (N)<br>(e) Incontinence chart (N) |
| 6 Faecal impaction | (i) Urinary incontinence<br>(ii) Spurious diarrhoea | (a) Enemas (N)<br>(b) Appropriate laxatives (D) |
| 7 Conflict with wife | (i) Institutionalisation<br>(ii) Neglect of patient after discharge<br>(iii) Violence to wife | (a) Prompt appropriate assistance (all services)<br>(b) Counselling (SW)<br>(c) Talking through problems (all personnel)<br>(d) Continuing support after discharge (HV or SW)<br>(e) Assurance of prompt assistance if things go wrong again (all services and out-patient clinics) |

Key: D = Doctor; SW = Social worker; N = Nurse; S = Surgeon; PT = Physiotherapist; HV = Health visitor;
OT = Occupational therapist.

## 4   Female, aged 83 years

**History**   This patient had suddenly developed severe back pain which had caused her to take to her bed. Home care in her warden-supervised flat had become very difficult when she became incontinent of urine. Treatment with simple analgesics had not relieved her pain.

She was seen at home and further questioning revealed she had been extremely fit until her recent illness. She became breathless if she walked quickly up an incline and complained that her bowels moved only every other day. Apart from these there had been no symptoms and she had been completely self-sufficient, doing all her own shopping, cooking and housework.

**Examination**   She was alert and looked well-nourished, and apart from considerable tenderness over her lumbar vertebrae there was little abnormal to find. However, vaginal examination revealed a hard nodular mass in the region of the uterine cervix.

She was admitted to hospital for further investigation which revealed an elevated erythrocyte sedimentation rate of 82 mm in one hour (Westergren) an elevated alkaline phosphatase of 232 international units/l, and an abnormal X-ray of her lumbar vertebrae which showed generalised bone rarefaction associated with collapse of the 2nd and 3rd lumbar vertebral bodies. A bone scan demonstrated areas of increased isotope uptake in her 2nd, 3rd and 5th lumbar vertebrae and in the shaft of her left femur.

Further examination by a gynaecologist under general anaesthesia confirmed a hard nodular mass around the uterine cervix which was involving the surrounding tissues. A biopsy confirmed the presence of an adenocarcinoma (Chapter 15: *malignancy*).

**Management**   The immediate problem was the relief of the severe back pain (Chapter 15: *relief of symptoms*), which was managed by giving her Buprenorphine 200 micrograms (sublingually) six-hourly. A radiotherapist was also consulted who felt that a course of radiotherapy to the primary tumour and to the secondaries might be effective in controlling symptoms. The combination of analgesia and radiotherapy controlled her pain but she remained drowsy, apathetic and incontinent.

During several short discussions with her it became apparent that she was aware of the diagnosis and outcome (Chapter 15: *what to tell the patient*). Communication between medical and nursing staff and the hospital chaplain was effective in providing her with reassurance and allaying anxiety about the distress likely to be involved in the terminal phase of her illness.

Over the next two weeks her condition continued to deteriorate. Her pain increased and it was necessary to give her morphine, adjusting the dose, sufficient to relieve her pain. She became increasingly drowsy and eventually developed a bronchopneumonia. Since this did not appear to be distressing her it was not treated with antibiotics (Chapter 5: *to treat or not to treat?*). She died 24 hours later.

SUMMARY

| Medical problems (diagnosis) | Possible effects | Possible actions |
|---|---|---|
| 1 Back pain | (i) Mobility | (a) Identify cause. NB importance of thorough physical examination. This can often save a lot of expensive and distressing laboratory investigations (D) |
| | (ii) Distress | (b) Treat with *small* but *regular* doses of analgesics (D) |
| 2 Carcinoma of cervix | Distress mainly due to secondaries | In view of metastases, give palliative therapy (D) |
| 3 Bony secondaries | Back pain | Consider radiotherapy if pain is severe (D) |
| 4 Anxiety | | (a) Talk through problems and fears (D, N, C, SW) |
| | | (b) Pass information to each other (D, N, C, SW) |
| | | (c) Consider tranquillisers (D) |
| 5 Immobility | (i) Pressure areas | (a) Provide good basic nursing care, eg. regular turning (N) |
| | (ii) Bronchopneumonia | (b) Only treat infection or venous thrombosis if they are causing distress (D) |
| | (iii) Venous thrombosis | |
| | (iv) Pulmonary embolism | |

*Key:* D = *Doctor;* C = *Chaplain;* N = *Nurse;* SW = *Social worker.*

## 5 Female, aged 89 years

**History** This patient was originally referred to the geriatric service three years previously when she was an in-patient with a fracture of the left hip (Chapter 7: *trauma*). At that time there seemed to be no barrier to discharge home so long as she regained sufficient mobility; she achieved this, but after returning home she complained of pain on walking and was readmitted under orthopaedic care and had a hip replacement operation.

She was next referred a year later as it was felt that she was failing to care for herself adequately because of immobility due to pain on walking. She was offered a place in a residential home, but refused and continued to live at home supported by community services and help from her relatives (Chapter 4: *physical disability*). Her final referral came eighteen months later. This time she was described as an elderly isolate who had been living alone for a long time. From time to time she took to her bed, and during these spells required home nursing care; after about a week she would get up and could then potter about her bungalow. However, on this occasion she had been in bed for 4 weeks, during which time she had been persistently incontinent of urine. The home nurses were visiting her three to four times a day but in spite of this were unable to give her adequate care. She was pyrexial, generally unwell, somewhat confused and getting dehydrated. A short admission to hospital was requested.

**Examination** She was visited at home, where examination confirmed the incontinence and revealed a respiratory tract infection which was probably the cause of her confusional state. Hospital admission was obviously urgently needed but she refused it. The only remaining course of action was to refer her case to the District Community Physician who arranged for her to be admitted under a magistrate's court order (Chapter 4: *attitudes in relation to social problems*).

**Management** On admission she was found to have evidence of a right lower-lobe pneumonia (Chapter 11: *pneumonia*), congestive cardiac failure (Chapter 10: *congestive cardiac failure*), faecal impaction (Chapter 14: *faecal impaction*), bilateral cataracts (Chapter 6: *cataract*), bilateral blepharitis and mental confusion (Chapter 9: *acute brain failure*). With the appropriate treatment she made a slow recovery and although she did not co-operate with the remedial therapists, she gradually became independent of help.

Her further care was discussed with her sister and niece who had been helping to look after her at home and with the social worker who had been supervising her case (Chapter 4: *attitudes in relation to social problems*), and it rapidly became apparent that the patient was an expert manipulator of people and situations (Chapter 4: *difficult personalities*). She had had three husbands, and was very careful with money, being regarded as a miser, but in spite of this liked to drink sherry (a bottle at a time) whenever she could get the opportunity. All concerned agreed that she ought to live in some form of residential accommodation, but she refused this advice and insisted on going home to live by herself (Chapter 4: *attitudes in relation to social problems*). After discussion with her general practitioner it was agreed that this must be allowed and she finally returned home after a two-month hospital admission.

Follow-up a year later found her managing well with the support of social services and the health care team (Chapter 5: *adjustment of the environment*).

SUMMARY

| Medical problems (diagnosis) | Possible effects | Possible actions |
|---|---|---|
| 1 Old fracture of hip | (i) Reduced mobility<br>(ii) Loss of self-care ability<br>(iii) Confinement to bed<br><br>(iv) Complications of bed rest | (a) Physiotherapy (PT)<br>(b) Day hospital care (D, N, OT, PT, SW)<br>(c) Rehabilitation as in-patient (D, N, OT, PT, SW)<br>(d) Admission for residential care (D) |
| 2 Lobar pneumonia | (i) Confusion<br>(ii) Incontinence<br>(iii) Dehydration<br>(iv) Venous thrombosis<br>(v) Pressure sores<br>(vi) Cardiac failure<br>(vii) Faecal impaction | (a) Antibiotics (D)<br>(b) Oxygen (D)<br>(c) Hospital admission (D, N) |
| 3 Congestive cardiac failure | (i) Confusion<br>(ii) Venous thrombosis | (a) Treat chest infection (D)<br>(b) Give diuretics with potassium (D) |
| 4 Dehydration | (i) Confusion<br>(ii) Venous thrombosis<br>(iii) Uraemia | (a) Give oral fluids (N)<br>(b) Give parenteral fluids (D) |
| 5 Faecal impaction | (i) Restlessness<br>(ii) Faecal incontinence<br>(iii) Urinary incontinence<br>(iv) Sub-acute obstruction | (a) Enema (N)<br>(b) Laxatives (D, N) |
| 6 Mental confusion | Loss of self-care ability | Treat 2, 3, 4 and 5 |

| Medical problems (diagnosis) | Possible effects | Possible actions |
|---|---|---|
| 7 Cataracts | (i) Confusion<br>(ii) Depression<br>(iii) Loss of self-care ability<br>(iv) Loss of balance | Refer to ophthalmologist |
| 8 Personality disorder | Strain on relatives and community services | (a) Accept less than ideal situation<br>(b) Meals-on-wheels (SW)<br>(c) Home help (SW)<br>(d) District nurse<br>(e) Follow-up (D, N, SW) |

*Key:* D = *Doctor;* N = *Nurse;* OT = *Occupational therapist;* PT = *Physiotherapist;* SW = *Social worker.*

## 6  Female, aged 65 years

**History**  This lady was referred because her husband found it difficult both to look after her and to do his job. The problem was one of gradual mental deterioration over a period of 7 years (Chapter 4: *mental disability*; Chapter 9: *chronic brain failure*), which had become much worse in the previous year as she had become totally disorientated in time and space. Her husband was able to converse with her and she retained a sense of humour, but she had not been out of the house unaccompanied for two years as she tended to get lost and to cross main roads without looking.

**Examination**  No physical abnormality was revealed, and special investigations were also negative, apart from the electroencephalographic tracing, which was compatible with degenerative brain changes (Chapter 9: *diagnosis*). Diagnosis, therefore, seemed to be one of dementia, probably due to Alzheimer's disease (Chapter 9: *aetiology*).

In the past she had had a Manchester repair for a prolapse (Chapter 14: *incontinence surgery*), a hiatus hernia and oesophagitis (Chapter 12: *hiatus hernia*), as well as chronic duodenal ulceration (Chapter 12: *peptic ulcers*). Four years before she was seen she had been admitted with obstructive jaundice which was thought to be due to chlorpromazine sensitivity (Chapter 12: *jaundice*). Gallstones (Chapter 12: *gallbladder disease*) were found on investigation but there was no evidence to suggest that these had caused her jaundice.

**Management**  Her husband said he was willing to continue to look after her if day care could be provided. Arrangements were made for her to attend an old people's home as a day patient, her husband taking her there in the morning and fetching her in the evening (Chapter 9: *management*). This arrangement worked extremely satisfactorily for 2 years, but her condition gradually deteriorated and she became more confused and liable to wander so that her care in an ordinary old people's home became impossible.

Since her husband did not wish her to be admitted to a long-stay psychogeriatric unit he made arrangements to give up his job and retire in order to look after his wife. As this was a full-time job, arrangements were made to take the patient regularly to a day hospital and short-term inpatient admissions were organised on an 'as required' basis to give him holidays and relief. While retirement meant loss of income to the husband this was to some extent compensated for by the wife being eligible for an attendance allowance. If this was inadequate the husband would also have been able to apply for an invalid care allowance (Chapter 4: *community services*).

SUMMARY

| Medical problems (diagnosis) | Possible effects | Possible action |
| --- | --- | --- |
| 1 Alzheimer's disease | (i) Wandering<br>(ii) Difficulty with self-care activities<br>(iii) Danger in house | (a) Day care (SW)<br>(b) Hospital relief admission (D)<br>(c) Permanent admission to hospital (D, N, OT, SW)<br>(d) Husband gives up job (SW)<br>(e) Support from psychiatric nurse |
| 2 Gallstones | (i) Acute cholecystitis<br>(ii) Obstructive jaundice<br>(iii) Cancer of gallbladder | (a) Remove gallbladder (D)<br>(b) Leave well alone (D) |
| 3 Duodenal ulcer | (i) Dyspepsia<br>(ii) Perforation<br>(iii) Haematemesis<br>(iv) Anaemia | (a) Since no symptoms, requires no treatment at present (D)<br>(b) Check haemoglobin (D) |
| 4 Hiatus hernia | (i) Chest pain<br>(ii) Dysphagia<br>(iii) Anaemia | Since no symptoms, requires no treatment at present (D) |
| 5 Husband out at work | Lack of support for patient | (a) See 1<br>(b) If 1(d) then husband applies for Invalid Care Allowance |

Key: D = Doctor; SW = Social worker; N = Nurse; OT = Occupational therapist.

## 7  Female, aged 100 years

**History**  This old lady was referred because her continuing care at home was placing an increasing strain upon her family. Until two months earlier she had been fairly independent, living upstairs and being able to wash, dress and make tea, but she had since then become gradually weaker, complaining of diarrhoea which was associated with loss of appetite and a feeling of nausea. She had had this complaint intermittently over the previous twenty years, following an abdominal operation, details of which were not available. She had lived with her son and daughter-in-law for 37 years, and the burden of her care over this time was now proving too much and was causing marital strife. This was probably accentuated by the fact that her only son was handicapped following a cerebral thrombosis, and consequently the burden of both husband and mother-in-law fell wholly on the wife (Chapter 4: *physical disability*).

**Examination**  Physical examination revealed a sprightly old lady who had a smooth red tongue, alopecia (baldness), an easily palpable abdominal aorta, mild ankle oedema and an ejection systolic murmur audible in both the aortic and mitral areas of the heart. Her liver was just palpable but otherwise there was no abnormality. In view of the loss of appetite it was felt that sub-nutrition could be contributing to her symptoms and a dietary assessment was made. Her calorie intake was approximately 1,000 K cal/day. She ate about 35 g of protein, 400 mg of calcium and took in 25 mg of vitamin C (Chapter 6: *poor nutrition*).

**Management**  Further investigations showed that she was anaemic, had a raised erythrocyte sedimentation rate and low blood levels of potassium, albumin, calcium and iron (Chapter 3: *haematological tests; biochemical tests*). Her serum alkaline phosphatase was elevated. An X-ray of her pelvis showed no evidence of osteomalacia but there were gross changes due to Paget's disease (Chapter 7: *Paget's disease of bone*). These multiple deficiencies were treated with iron and vitamin D supplements.

A barium meal examination showed an abnormal bowel pattern which was compatible with a diagnosis of malabsorption (Chapter 12: *malabsorption*); it also showed small bowel diverticula. Since bacterial overgrowth in small bowel diverticula was a likely cause of malabsorption and diarrhoea she was put onto doxycyclin, and on this *régime* her diarrhoea settled.

The question was raised of the extent of investigation. In fact, relatively simple blood tests and X-rays were not in themselves too distressing for the patient, even at her great age, and enabled a reasonable assessment of her clinical state to be made, thereby allowing a rational and effective treatment programme to be initiated (Chapter 3: *how much is justified?*).

This was successful in that she remained well and asymptomatic for almost a year following her discharge.

As her son and daughter-in-law were unwilling to take her home she was discharged to a local authority old people's home where she remains well (Chapter 4: *residential accommodation*). This solution was discussed with the patient herself, who agreed that it was appropriate before it was implemented (Chapter 4: *attitudes in relation to social problems*).

SUMMARY

| Medical problems (diagnosis) | Possible effects | Possible actions |
|---|---|---|
| 1 Extreme old age | Slight reduction in mobility | (a) Increasing support to relatives (SW) <br> (b) Residential care (SW) |
| 2 Low dietary intake | (i) Anaemia <br> (ii) Osteomalacia | Iron and vitamin D supplements (D) |
| 3 Small bowel diverticula | (i) Malabsorption <br> (ii) Osteomalacia | Antibiotics (D) |
| 4 Paget's disease | (i) Nil <br> (ii) Cardiac failure <br> (iii) Bone pain <br> (iv) Fractures <br> (v) Deafness | Since no symptoms no treatment necessary (D) |
| 5 Elderly and disabled relatives | Inability to cope with patient | (a) Increasing support to relatives by primary care teams and day centre <br> (b) Residential care (SW) |

*Key:* D = *Doctor;* SW = *Social worker.*

## 8 Male, aged 73 years

**History** This patient was referred from a residential home. The main problem was that since admission there had been a deterioration in his mobility so that he required help with walking and even with this he was having recurrent falls (Chapter 8: *falls*). He also had difficulty in washing and dressing himself, and over the last two weeks had become incontinent of both urine and faeces.

There was a long history of a poor memory punctuated with outbursts of aggression. Indeed, this problem had made it impossible for his elderly wife to cope and had resulted in his admission to residential care two months prior to his referral to the geriatric unit (Chapter 9: *brain failure*).

In the past he had been troubled by a cough associated with a clear sputum, and he had been treated for swollen ankles. Tuberculous glands had been excised from his neck in childhood.

His wife's physical health was good, but there had been marital problems for many years. With the deterioration in his mental function, life at home had consisted of persistent rows, and eventually it had been decided that the only practical solution was to admit him to residential care.

His drug treatment consisted of frusemide 40 mg daily; Slow K 600 mg three times daily; salbutamol 2 mg 6-hourly; thioridazine 50 mg at night; quinine sulphate 600 mg at night; and danthron 10 ml as required.

**Examination** He had a rigid facial expression. There was a scar on the left side of his neck, and purpuric patches on both forearms. All four limbs were rigid, and he had a tremor of his tongue and arms which was most marked when he was at rest. When he was persuaded to stand he leant forward and walked with shuffling steps. His pulse was regular, his lying blood pressure 140/90 mmHg and his standing one 110/80 mmHg. There was a trace of ankle oedema. His abdomen was rather distended and his rectum loaded with hard faeces. A mental test score suggested only moderate cognitive impairment, but his behaviour during the interview suggested some degree of depression.

**Management** All his drugs were discontinued. Following this, however, there was an increase in ankle oedema and he was put on bendrofluazide 10 mg daily with Slow K 600 mg three times daily. Discontinuation of drugs was followed by narrowing of the gap between his lying and standing blood pressure. There was no deterioration in his behaviour when sedation was discontinued. Indeed, he became more alert and more cooperative (Chapter 5: *treatment and management*).

He was treated with increasing doses of levodopa and benserazide which reduced his rigidity and tremor. He also became much more cheerful. He remained immobile, however, and this only improved after a

6-week course of physiotherapy which concentrated on improving the size of his steps. During this time an occupational therapist gave him training in washing and dressing. As a result of this, he was able to walk with a Zimmer frame, and wash, dress and toilet himself (Chapter 8: *the neurology of old age*).

His faecal impaction was cleared with three phosphate enemas in the week after admission, and his bowel function regulated with regular doses of bran. It was hoped that this would also reduce his urinary incontinence, but unfortunately it persisted, and cystometry therefore was performed: this showed that he had a hypertonic bladder, which responded to propantheline in a dose of 15 mg three times daily (Chapter 14: *incontinence*).

The social worker had a long discussion with his wife, but it became clear that a reconciliation was most unlikely. It was decided, therefore, to discharge him back to residential care. Arrangements were made for him to be followed up at the day hospital.

SUMMARY

| Medical problems (diagnosis) | Possible effects | Possible actions |
|---|---|---|
| 1 Parkinson's disease | (i) Limited mobility<br>(ii) Mental impairment<br>(iii) Depression<br>(iv) Postural hypotension | (a) Drug treatment (D)<br>(b) Mobilisation (PT, N)<br>(c) ADL training (OT) |
| 2 Alzheimer's disease | (i) Aggression | (a) Stop inappropriate medication (D)<br>(b) Counsel wife (SW)<br>(c) Admit to institutional care (SW) |
| 3 Congestive cardiac failure | (i) Ankle oedema | (a) Treat with diuretics (but make sure of diagnosis first) (D) |
| 4 Urinary incontinence | (i) Long stay hospital care | (a) Investigate cause (D, N)<br>(b) Toilet training (N)<br>(c) Stop diuretics (D)<br>(d) Give anticholinergic agents (D) |
| 5 Faecal impaction | (i) Spurious diarrhoea<br>(ii) Urinary incontinence<br>(iii) Agitation | (a) Enema (D, N)<br>(b) Bran (D, N) |
| 6 Marital strife | (i) Aggression<br>(ii) Refusal to accept home | (a) Counselling (SW)<br>(b) Improve medical problems (D, N, OT, PT) |

Key: D = Doctor; N = Nurse; PT = *Physiotherapist*; OT = *Occupational therapist*; SW = *Social worker*.

## 9 Male, aged 88 years

**History** This man had taken to his bed following the onset of a bout of watery diarrhoea several days previously. There had been evidence of some mental impairment for a considerable time, but he had become much more confused with the onset of the diarrhoea. Diabetes had been diagnosed several years previously and this had been treated with tolbutamide 500 mg twice daily. Despite this he had developed a proliferative retinopathy and had been registered as being partially sighted. He also had had congestive cardiac failure and this was being treated currently with digoxin 62.5 mcg daily. There was a past history of appendicitis 5 years previously, and reduction of an obstructed inguinal hernia 6 years previously.

He lived in a bungalow across the road from his daughter and son-in-law. Unfortunately, he had stubbornly refused to allow her in to help with cooking or housework. As a result the house had become dilapidated, dirty and untidy.

**Examination** He was pleasant but very muddled. His tongue was dry and his skin lax and inelastic. His pulse had a rate of 100/min, was regular and was of low volume, and his blood pressure 110/80 mmHg when lying and 60/40 mmHg when standing. There were no abnormal signs in his chest, and the only abnormal signs on his abdomen were the scars of previous surgery. Both retinae showed signs of a proliferative retinopathy. The only biochemical abnormality was moderate elevation of his blood urea concentration. His random blood glucose concentration was within normal limits.

**Management** All drug treatment was stopped. Following this his diarrhoea settled, and his confusion resolved. It then emerged that he had been taking a tablet of saccharin first thing in the morning, and putting three tablets of digoxin in every cup of tea which he had. When his blood glucose concentration was rechecked several days after admission it was found to be marginally elevated. He was put back on tolbutamide in a dose of 500 mg daily (Chapter 13: *homeostasis*).

His blood urea fell, his postural hypotension resolved and he regained his mobility. He also was able to wash and dress himself. The occupational therapist, however, found that he was unable to perform satisfactorily in the kitchen. In view of this, of his problem with medication, and of the difficulty his family had in getting access to his house, it was decided to persuade him to move into residential care. Surprisingly, he seemed pleased with the suggestion. His house therefore was sold and he was settled in a private residential home within easy reach of his family.

SUMMARY

| Medical problems (diagnosis) | Possible effects | Possible actions |
|---|---|---|
| 1 Diarrhoea | (i) Faecal incontinence | (a) Treat with codeine etc. (D) |
| | (ii) Dehydration | (b) Stop digoxin (D) |
| | (iii) Confusion | |
| 2 Dehydration | (i) Confusion | (a) Control cause (D) |
| | (ii) Immobility | (b) Push oral fluids (N) |
| | (iii) Postural hypotension | |
| 3 Digoxin toxicity | (i) Confusion | (a) Stop digoxin (D) |
| | (ii) Diarrhoea | (b) Train in self medication (OT, N) |
| | (iii) Cardiotoxicity | (c) Supervise medication at home (HV, DN) |
| 4 Congestive cardiac failure | (i) Inappropriate medication in condition which has resolved | (a) Review necessity for continued medication |
| 5 Diabetes mellitus | (i) Confusion due to hyperglycaemia | (a) Regularly monitor blood glucose (D) |
| | (ii) Confusion due to overtreatment | (b) Give appropriate hypo- glycaemia in appropriate dose (D) |
| | (iii) Retinopathy | |
| 6 Postural hypotension | (i) Immobility | (a) Correct dehydration (D) |
| | (ii) Falls | (b) Mobilise (N, PT) |
| 7 Self neglect | (i) Subnutrition | (a) Increase support at home (R, HH, SW, MW) |
| | (ii) Poor drug compliance | (b) Increase supervision at home (R, HV) |
| | (iii) Hypothermia | (c) Arrange residential care (R, SW) |
| | (iv) Safety hazard | |
| 8 Visual impairment | (i) Falls | (a) Put on Blind Register and organise appropriate services (SW) |
| | (ii) Poor self care capacity | |

*Key:* D = *Doctor;* N = *Nurse;* OT = *Occupational therapist;* PT = *Physiotherapist;*
SW = *Social worker;* R = *Relative;* HH = *Home help;* HV = *Health visitor;*
DN = *District nurse;* MW = *Meals-on-wheels service.*

# CHAPTER 1

# Demography and Population Statistics

The sudden rapid increase in the proportion of old people in society seems to be a relatively recent phenomenon. The process has been quietly simmering since prehistory, but the full impact has only become apparent in the present century (Fig. 1.1). The so-called developed nations have the highest proportions of old people, but it is important to realise that the elderly in Africa, Latin America and South East Asia will be the fastest growing of any age group (including children) between 1985 and 2000. Thus, in these regions, the number of people over the age of 60 years will increase during these 15 years by more than 100%.

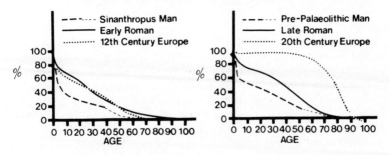

Figure 1.1   Survival curves through the ages

This change in population structure is not due to the old living longer, but rather to fewer young and middle-aged people dying. Figure 1.2 differentiates, in a statistical way, between premature deaths due to accidents and disease, and senescent deaths due to inevitable ageing. Modern medicine, public health, better nutrition, social improvements, and so on, have reduced the premature mortality rate with little effect on the senescent mortality rate. Thus, life expectancy at birth for a boy is now nearly 70 years in the United Kingdom – this represents an increase of

27

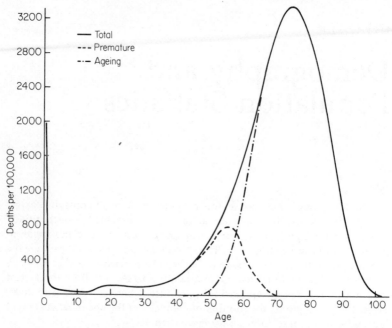

Figure 1.2   Curve of deaths, English Life Table 13, 1970–72; men (OPCS 1980)

more than 21 years (45%) over the course of this century. Over the same period the remaining life expectancy for a 65 year old man has increased by approximately one year (8%) to 12.2 years. It is likely that the phenomenon of increasing life expectancy at birth brought about by medical and social 'engineering' is subject to the law of diminishing returns. Thus, if a 'cure for cancer' became available and no individual died from any form of this disease, the increase in average life expectancy in a developed nation would be hardly measurable. The survival curve (Fig. 1.1) is now almost rectilinear.

By the turn of this century, the *world* population of people over the age of 60 years will have reached 580 million, a 60% increase over 25 years, and two-thirds of these individuals will live in the *less-developed* regions of the world. Thus, by the year 2000, very nearly one in ten individuals world-wide will be over 60 years of age. The economic and social consequences will be no less important than the implications for Health Service planning and provision, but it is only the latter aspects which are examined here. Figure 1.3 shows the changes in population structure of the United Kingdom which have occurred since the beginning of the

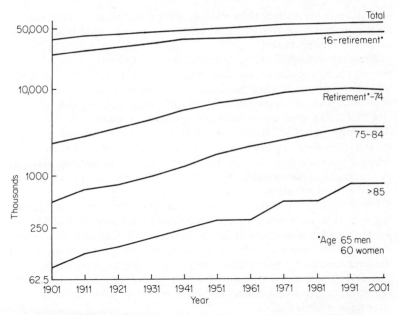

Figure 1.3   Age structure of the population 1901–2001, United Kingdom
(OPCS 1980)

century and provides best estimates forward to the next century. It can be
seen that from the 1950s the main growth segment has been in the elderly
population. Over the course of the next 20 years the number of people
over the age of 65 will increase by a modest 4%. However, within this
population the greatest growth in numbers will occur in the oldest group.
Thus, the over 75s will increase by 18%, but the over 85s will increase by
twice as much – 38%.

## Health of the elderly

Most elderly people are healthy in both mind and body, and even into
extreme old age they are able to manage an independent, unsupported
way of life. They should be encouraged and, if need be, assisted to continue in this way. Indeed, to a certain extent, only the fit survive and
extremely elderly individuals could be considered the 'biological elite' of
the human species. The social rôle of the elderly depends upon the society, the culture and the individual. There is no doubt that the elderly were
held in higher esteem in the past than in present day societies, although

even now we are content to let 80-year-olds run our political lives, control nuclear weapons, or allocate health resources, whilst forbidding 65-year-olds from driving buses!

While physiological ageing does lead to some decline in physical, mental and social capacities, the degree is not usually significant until the system is perturbed, when the diminished reserve capacity of the elderly individual becomes apparent. Some old people adopt a negative life cycle (Fig. 1.4), and may go on to develop a sick or dependent rôle. This descending spiral of diminishing ability may be reinforced by well-meaning relatives or even some caring professionals (Chapter 4). A positive life cycle (Fig. 1.5) for the elderly requires excitement, risk and even danger. It also requires the recognition of this fact by health professionals and society generally.

Unfortunately, ill-health, disease and disability increase with increasing age – this is not entirely surprising if one considers that most diseases are the result of some form of interaction between man and his environment, and the longer an individual has been exposed to risk, the higher the probability of a pernicious interaction. There have been few comprehensive and detailed health surveys of old people, but all those reported confirm an exponential increase in disease with increasing age, starting in middle life.

In general terms, approximately 15% of the United Kingdom population is over the age of 65 years. Thus, in a standard population of 10,000 individuals of all ages, 1,500 will be over the age of 65 years, and of these

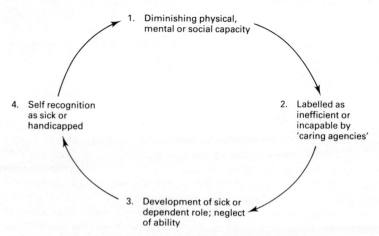

Figure 1.4   The negative life cycle: a vicious circle of ill health in the elderly

only 66 (4.4%) will be in an institution (hospital, nursing home or old people's home) at any one time. The vast majority (95.6%) of old people live in the community. However, within the population of old people

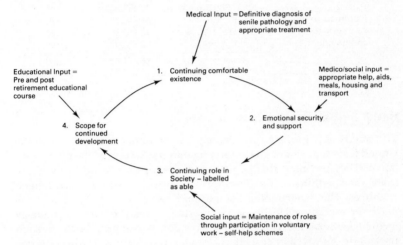

Figure 1.5   The positive life cycle: the maintenance of good health in the elderly

there is a marked age-related institutionalisation rate. Thus, nearly half of all individuals over 95 years of age are in institutions at any one time. The proportion of old people in institutions also varies considerably from country to country, and indeed within countries. In the United Kingdom approximately half of the institutionalised elderly are in hospital, while the remainder are equally divided between private nursing and public (Local Authority OPH) accommodation – the latter, in the main, not providing skilled nursing support.

Every health service has difficulty matching resources to need, not primarily because of financial constraints, although these are obviously important, but rather to lack of hard data. In Table 1.1 an attempt has been made to relate disability (not need) to accommodation. It is obvious that two-thirds of the most severely disabled and dependent individuals (bedfast) are not in hospital, but in the community. Excluding these individuals, a further 300 old people have significantly impaired mobility, either physically or mentally determined, and again the majority of these live at home. These figures are generalised aggregates and each area needs to collect such information if it is to plan and to provide a service for old people. Equally, planning requires coordination of both hospital and community – neither can plan or work in isolation.

Table 1.1  Disability and Residence: 1,500 People Over the Age of 65 Years

| Functional Level | Home | Institution | Total |
|---|---|---|---|
| Bedfast | 29 (63.0%) | 17 (37.0%) | 46 |
| Confined to 'house' | 158 (91.9%) | 14 (8.1%) | 172 |
| Mobile with aid | 115 (89.8%) | 13 (10.2%) | 128 |
| Independent | 1,132 (98.1%) | 22 (1.9%) | 1,154 |
| | 1,434 (95.8%) | 66 (4.4%) | 1,500 |

## Health services for the elderly (Fig. 1.6)

The elderly account for approximately half of all hospital facilities in the United Kingdom, although comprising only 15 per cent of the total population. They consume about one quarter of all prescribed drugs and use more than a third of the primary care teams' (general practitioners) resources. The demographic changes outlined previously account in the main for escalating Health Service costs – the use of high technology medicine may be individually expensive but used appropriately, even in the elderly, may well be cost effective in terms of early diagnosis, effective treatment, and prevention or amelioration of dependency and disability.

## Community care

The successful management of an ill, elderly patient depends upon a rapid response from the primary health care team – delay in meeting his medical needs can lead to accelerated physical, mental or social deterioration, and to the development of semi-permanent dependency. The difficulties of accurate clinical diagnosis and evaluation are outlined throughout this book. This, however, is not to deny the skilled rôle of other health professionals in the primary health care team. Thus, as can be seen from the case histories, the district nurse, health visitor and social worker all have very important parts to play in the location, overall management and skilled support and treatment of ill old people. The primary health care team needs to be led by a skilled doctor, for the early diagnosis and management of ill-health in the elderly cannot be delegated to non-physicians.

One problem of particular moment with the elderly in the community is the phenomenon of unreported ill-health. Old people tend to be stoical in their acceptance of disease and increasing disability. This attitude may also be reinforced, unfortunately, by well-meaning relatives who attribute symptoms and signs of disease in the elderly to old age rather than to disease (Chapter 6). It is important that this iceberg of disease, most of it entirely treatable at an early stage, be uncovered by the primary health care team. In order to carry this out, each practitioner needs to have an

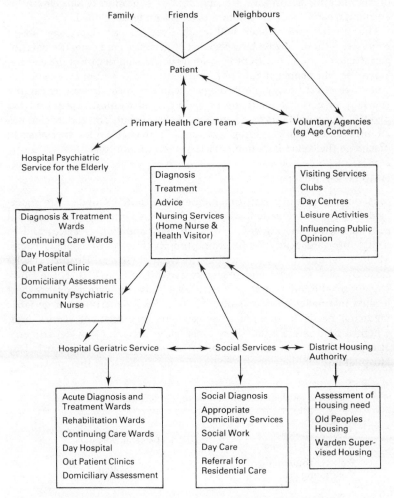

Figure 1.6   Hospital and community services for the elderly

age/sex register which can readily be obtained (and free of charge) from the Health Service administration in the United Kingdom (Family Practitioner Committee). Using this register, patients 'at risk' can be listed so that they may be kept under observation by the health visitor or the district nurse. Patients may also be screened, although the value of screening as opposed to 'case finding' is doubtful. Nevertheless, the earlier symptomatic ill-health can be treated the higher the probability of maintaining health and activity. Health education of the elderly to encourage early medical attention is as yet underdeveloped.

The general practitioner will often need to call upon specialised resources – these may be the specialist in geriatric medicine, the psychogeriatrician or other health professional specialising in care of the elderly. However, old people should not be disenfranchised from other specialisms such as cardiology, nephrology, respirology, etc. In no way can the specialty of geriatric medicine provide overall medical care for all old people – nor would this be a beneficial development. The geriatrician has an important rôle in providing back-up skills to enable other specialists to discharge their elderly patients back to the community.

## Hospital services

Most departments of geriatric medicine in the United Kingdom are organised on progressive patient care lines. Basically each department should provide acute assessment wards, a rehabilitation service and a continuing-care facility. To function properly the Department of Geriatric Medicine should be located within the District General Hospital (DGH) close by all diagnostic and treatment facilities (Table 1.2). Some slow-stream rehabilitation and probably all continuing-care beds are best located in smaller units outside the DGH. Each department of geriatric medicine needs to provide a comprehensive outpatient service and, where appropriate, a domiciliary consultative service. Many departments also provide an outpatient rehabilitation service using a Geriatric Day Hospital or even develop domiciliary teams of remedial therapists.

Table 1.2   Recommended Norms for Geriatric Hospital Services

| Geriatric Beds | | |
|---|---|---|
| Acute assessment | 3 ⎫ | |
| Quick rehabilitation | 2 ⎬ | District General Hospital |
| Slow rehabilitation | 2 ⎫ | |
| Continuing care | 3 ⎬ | Community Hospital |
| | 10/1,000 elderly | |
| Psychiatric beds | 3 | |
| Joint psychogeriatric beds | 0.5–0.8 | |
| Geriatric day hospital places | 2 | per 1,000 elderly |
| Psychiatric day hospital places | 2–3 | |
| Local Authority residential beds | 25 | |

*Acute assessment.* All patients should have the benefit of a full medical work-up (Chapters 2 and 3). Certainly, no elderly patient should be accepted for long-term care either within hospital or even within the community without this initial investigation. The only difference between an acute assessment ward in a department of geriatric medicine and a general or internal medical ward is the greater emphasis on functional aspects of disability within the geriatric area. In both types of ward the medical diagnosis, treatment and clinical management should be identical. The vast majority of old people admitted to an acute assessment ward should come from the community and be returned there well within one month.

*Rehabilitation.* A number of old people admitted to acute geriatric or, indeed, to any medical or surgical ward will, after treatment of their acute precipitating condition, require further physical rehabilitation. This is best carried out within a suitable environment orientated towards the slower progress of such individuals. Rehabilitation patients do not do well in the environment of an acute ward admitting patients at all times of the day and night. The medical management of patients in rehabilitation wards needs to be continued but now the emphasis should be more on physical therapy. For this a fully-trained team of integrated remedial therapists (physiotherapists, occupational therapists, speech therapists) is required. The ward nurses also are important components of any rehabilitation programme and need to work closely with the therapists in a coordinated plan. In this environment the old patient with, for example, a stroke (Chapter 8) can be retrained to maximise his potential abilities and overcome or adapt to his disabilities. In many cases this rehabilitation programme makes the difference between long-term institutional care and living with residual disability and maximum function in the community.

*Continuing care.* There are a number of individuals who, it must be accepted, do not respond to rehabilitation. In the main this is due to the extreme disability produced by a serious disease. Unfortunately, in a minority of cases this dependency may have been produced by the Health Service itself – either physicians were too slow to act at the initial presentation of the disease or even were unaware of the subtle signs of disease (Chapter 2) until too late. Such disabled individuals require long-term nursing support. This can best be accomplished outside the district general hospital which is orientated towards a rapid turnover of patients. Unfortunately, continuing-care patients within an acute hospital environment often get the label of failure attached to them with all its negative connotations. A small nursing unit, preferably located within the community it serves, requires adequate numbers of skilled nurses, therapists and activities organisers to provide a suitable environment which allows disabled individuals to maximise the quality of their remaining life.

*Psychogeriatric care.* Because of the high incidence of psychiatric disease in the elderly, each geriatric unit needs to work in close association with a psychiatrist with a special responsibility for the elderly or, preferably, a full-time psychogeriatrician. Ideally, the psychogeriatric and the geriatric units need to be in close geographical relationship within the district general hospital to allow cross consultation, joint management, and so on. It is important, however, not to allow a psychogeriatric service to become a dementia service. Affective disorders and neuroses are extremely common in the elderly, often coexisting with or being potentiated by physical disabilities, and their effective therapy can speed rehabilitation and develop independence, allowing early discharge back to the community. The close liaison between geriatric and psychogeriatric services may be accomplished by joint sharing of beds, although this is not uniformly essential. A psychogeriatrician with a team of community psychiatric nurses and social workers can provide a community back-up programme for the support of most patients and, more importantly, their relatives, even when the patient is severely disabled by chronic brain failure (Chapter 9).

Whilst the progressive patient care model is the commonest scheme of geriatric care in the United Kingdom, there are others. In some areas the geriatric service provides a comprehensive and exclusive medical service for all individuals over a certain age which is determined by the allocation of resources between general (internal) and geriatric medicine. In a few areas acute resources are shared equally between the two divisions, with the geriatrician playing a full part in a general medical service and, in addition, providing a geriatric rehabilitation and continuing-care service for the elderly. A final model, common in Scandinavia, is for the geriatrician to be a specialist in long-term continuing care, with no commitment to acute clinical work, nor even to rehabilitation.

All hospital care is expensive, but it should be realised that geriatric hospital care is extremely expensive on a case cost basis. For example, in 1972 it cost £79 for each obstetric/gynaecological patient, £91 for each ophthalmological or general surgical patient, £105 per general medical patient, £245 for a dermatological patient, £369 for nephrological, cardiological or neurological cases, and £391 for individual geriatric cases (RAWP, 1976). Perusal of the Health Service costing returns for 1982 suggest that these costs have now risen by a factor of 4.7. However, costs continue to rise and as can be seen from Table 1.3 the cost per geriatric patient case now exceeds £2,000.

Little wonder then that politicians blow trumpets for the community for, as Table 1.3 shows, the cost per patient case is about a third of the cost of a hospital case. We need, therefore, to reduce long stay hospital care for

Table 1.3   Costing Indicators

| Type of hospital | Cost per in-patient day | Cost per in-patient case |
|---|---|---|
| District General | £78.63 | £  671.00 |
| Acute Support | £72.37 | £  750.00 |
| Community | £50.14 | £  765.00 |
| Mainly Geriatric | £41.14 | £2,381.00 |
| Other non-psychiatric | £79.19 | £1,137.00 |
| Mental Handicap | £24.94 | — |
| Mental Illness | £31.16 | — |

*Source:* SW Thames RHA Financial Digest 1984 (Year to 31.3.84)

disabled and dependent old people to a minimum. If we are going to achieve this then disability must be prevented or ameliorated by expert medical and rehabilitation therapy or more disabled people should be looked after in their own homes. If this latter option is to be exploited as a national thrift measure, then it must be appreciated that the already heavy burden (Table 1.1) borne by relatives and other non-professionals will be increased. Without an appropriate response by the Health Service in resource allocation, then the whole concept of a swing away from hospital care is doomed to failure.

Institutional care of the disabled is cheaper outside hospitals than inside them. There are several reasons for this – firstly, the level of support (nursing) is much less as very few old people's homes (OPH) employ nurses, and, secondly, the residents themselves contribute directly to revenue costs of their own care. In 1976/77 over 30% of the total cost (£267,350,000) of Local Authority spending on old person's accommodation was actually paid for by the residents themselves. Finally, the 'hidden' costs of community care (rent, heating, etc., district nursing, voluntary support) are rarely involved in any accounting returns.

Similarly, it may be cheaper to care for the sick elderly in their own homes. Moreover, this may be in concordance with their own wishes. As a result different systems of care are evolving. Hospital teams are providing short-term care to the elderly at home, thereby supporting the primary care team. Hospital and social services are providing support to carers by taking the disabled elderly into the day hospital or day centres, or by providing holiday or even relief admission to long-stay hospitals or local authority old peoples' homes. Regular relief admission on a 'shared care' basis may also be adopted by agreement with carers as a method of care which is acceptable to all parties. In this way, long-stay places may be eked out so that one bed may serve three or four patients on a regular rota basis. Nevertheless, this puts an additional strain on hospital staff even if it helps to achieve a better use of resources.

## Further reading

*BMA Report of the Working Party on Services for the Elderly* (1976) British Medical Association

DHSS (Welsh Office) 1983 *Health Service Costing Returns for 1982*. London: HMSO

Harris A I & Buckle J R (1971) *Handicapped and Impaired in Great Britain*. London: HMSO

Kinnaird J, Brotherton Sir John & Williamson J (eds) (1981) *The Provision of Care for the Elderly*. Edinburgh: Churchill Livingstone

MacLennan W J (1976) The elderly in the community. *Update*, **13**, 1245–1252.

*Population Trends* (1982) London: HMSO

Resource Allocation Working Party (1976) *Sharing Resources for Health in England*. London: HMSO

Shanas F, Townsend P, Wedderburn D, Friis H, Milhøj P & Stehousner J (1968) *Old People in Three Industrial Societies*. London: Routledge & Kegan Paul

Shegog R F A (ed) (1981) *The Impending Crisis of Old Age. A Challenge to Ingenuity*. Nuffield Provincial Hospitals Trust, Oxford University Press

CHAPTER 2

# The Elderly Patient and His Clinical Problems

It has often been asked 'What is so different about the geriatric patient? He is only you or I a little older'. This is only true up to a point, for many differences do exist between the elderly patient and his younger counterparts.

## Admission to hospital

For many elderly patients, admission to a geriatric ward is their first experience of hospital, while in others their hospital experience may not have been for many years. Consequently, their knowledge and ideas of hospital may be totally false, being coloured by what they have heard or previously experienced. This applies particularly to patients coming into the geriatric ward, since this is often considered to be little more than the last resting place prior to death. The evolution of modern hospitals and their geriatric units from old workhouses to present day excellence within the life-time of local old people may not be fully appreciated by the elderly person referred to that hospital.

For these reasons patients require reassurance and a careful explanation of the function of the ward and what will happen to them. This condition will obviously be met if the consultant under whom a patient is to be admitted has seen him prior to his admission and explained the problems to him. If this does not happen, the task should be taken over by the general practitioner, the district nurse or the health visitor of the primary health care team, and patients being admitted from residential homes should have the problems explained to them by a member of the primary health care team, or by the matron, or their relatives. If a patient is to be transferred from another hospital ward an explanation should be given not only by the geriatric staff when they see the patient but also by the staff of the transferring ward. The latter should always make quite sure that the patient's relatives have also been told. Equally, for those patients being transferred for rehabilitation both patients and their relatives should be disabused of the notion that geriatric care equates with long-stay care.

The primary objective with any elderly patient admitted to the geriatric ward must be to enable him to resume his place in society and the community as quickly as possible, so the accent is on the rapid attainment of self-sufficiency. Since patients are encouraged to get up and dress as soon as possible, they should bring their clothes with them. Whenever possible, patients should be allowed to return to their homes at week-ends; five-days-a-week treatment and care experiments have already been performed with success.

## The elderly patient as an individual

With the elderly the doctor/nurse/patient relationship is different from that of any other group, for a gap of at least one and often three or four generations exists. Whereas the senior doctor is regarded as a father or companion figure by many of his patients, to the elderly he represents a son or a grandson. While it is very good for the ego of the 50-year-old professor to be addressed as 'boy', he and all others need to exhibit great tact and competence if they are to gain the confidence of the elderly patient. Since hospital staff are strangers they have an advantage in this respect, but they will be treated initially with great suspicion and must exercise caution and restraint in their management of the patient. There is no doubt that many elderly people are afraid of being 'mucked about' or 'experimented with' in hospital, but if the reasons for procedures are fully explained there are few patients who are more co-operative and reasonable. Generally speaking, the elderly patient is one of the most rewarding of all patients to treat, for his expectations of gain are low and he responds gratefully to care, patience and skilled attention.

In order to understand their patients, all hospital staff must have some knowledge of the ageing process and the type of person that the patient has been. Here the hospital doctor may be at a disadvantage when compared with the family doctor who has probably known the patient over many years. It is vital that those based in hospital ensure that they collect any relevant information from the family doctor. The following conversation took place one day. Nurse (on telephone to resident doctor): 'Dr Green, your patient Mrs Harris, who was admitted this afternoon, is terribly confused. Do you think you could come and write her up for a sedative?' Dr Green: 'How do you mean? Is she noisy?' Nurse: 'Yes! She is shouting and swearing at us, she has already hit one of the nurses, we can't get her undressed and she wants to go out and buy some cigarettes.'

From this brief conversation it might be concluded that the old lady was confused, aggressive and, to say the least, difficult. There is no doubt that the nurse/patient relationship was under considerable strain. Fortunately for the hospital and also for future doctor/nurse/patient relations, the resident on his way to the ward met the consultant who asked if Mrs Harris had yet been admitted. He went on to explain that she had come in for investigation of her anaemia, which had not responded to iron medication so that barium studies were considered to be necessary. Since she was 85 it had been decided that it was kinder to perform these investigations in hospital (Chapter 3: *where should investigations be done?*). The consultant further commented that she was a strong-willed, dominant old lady who smoked like a chimney and ruled her family with a rod of iron. On hearing the resident's story he laughed and said: 'Well has she got any cigarettes because she certainly won't settle down without them. Maybe she genuinely does want to go out and buy some.' They went together to the ward and sure enough this was the explanation for the old lady's apparently outrageous, confused behaviour. Doctor/patient relationships were excellent, therefore, right from the beginning, but it took a little longer to establish nurse/patient relationships!

As people age there is a tendency for them to become more rigid in their response to life and more set in their ways. Consequently simple routines become much more important and their omission or alteration can give rise to frustration, and sometimes confusion, in old people. Decision-making may also be more difficult and routine hospital administrative procedures prove obstacles to treatment; one example is the need to sign an anaesthetic consent form. It should also be recognised that these changes affect the ability of the elderly to give an accurate clinical history.

## Clinical history-taking

The elderly are just as capable of giving an account of their illness, complaints and problems as younger patients. However, for the above reasons the time sequence of events may be muddled and whoever obtains a history from an old person should always check it. Sources of confirmation include relatives, neighbours, general practitioner, social worker, other hospital staff and previous records. These difficulties make history-taking more time-consuming in the elderly than in the young.

## Problems of communication

These relate particularly to speech and hearing. Dysarthria and aphasia are common complications of neurological disease in old people. The advice of the speech therapist should be sought as soon as possible with regard to both aphasia and dysarthria, because assessment of the speech deficit is important and may be helped by aids such as pictures. The absence of teeth, and ill-fitting false teeth, are more easily remediable disabilities but so often overlooked.

Deafness is frequently denied by old people, but they will admit to being hard of hearing and they can often hear well if speech is clearly, slowly and loudly enunciated. Shouting is not only embarrassing but often unnecessary. When speaking to a deaf person it is important to position yourself so that he sees your face clearly, for he may have considerable lip reading ability. Deafness in the elderly is often due to the accumulation of wax in the ears. Removal of the wax may not be possible at the time of the initial examination and the recording of details may need to be postponed until this has been done. Hearing aids can be of considerable value in establishing easy communication. The speaking tube or ear trumpet is one type of hearing aid which may be of considerable use in the out-patient clinic or surgery and is invaluable in domiciliary work; being cheap, it should be part of the equipment of every doctor, nurse and social worker who has regular contact with old people (*cf.* Chapter 6).

## Special points to elicit from the older patient

One feature which often distinguishes the elderly patient from others is his limited capacity for self-care. Old people often depend on the help of others to maintain their place in the community, and this dependence may be due to old age alone or, more likely, to old age linked to disability. A patient's capacity to deal with his personal environment is of great importance. To quote a simple example, someone who is unable to climb stairs on account of breathlessness will be totally marooned if he lives in a second-floor flat which has no lift, but if he lives in a bungalow or a ground-floor flat in an area with level surroundings he may well be relatively independent. It is essential that this type of information be included in the case record.

The patient's insight into his capacity should be checked against the views of others (Chapter 9); these may include the general practitioner, the district nurse or other professional observers and relatives, friends and neighbours. It is quite common for different people to have different opinions about an individual's ability and what type of provision is necessary for his future care. A detailed social history which clearly states and distinguishes the view of the patient and others who have been concerned with his care in the community is of vital importance in reaching a rational and agreed decision about his further management. It saves a lot of time and is likely to solve the problem which most concerns the patient. Many of the more esoteric medical and social conditions which the professional worker uncovers may be of little importance.

### Social acceptability (Case 3)

A patient's history must record details of his behaviour and habits, because the ease or difficulty of his discharge will often depend on whether these are acceptable to others. While this information may be discovered by direct questioning of the patient, it is more likely to be obtained from those who have known him at home. The most striking example of a behavioural problem is incontinence, obviously a social barrier as well as an unpleasant state for the patient. A careful history is of vital importance in every case if the cause is to be discovered (*see* Chapter 4).

### Nutrition

The subject of nutrition is discussed in Chapter 6. A detailed dietary history is often difficult to obtain direct from the patient, but it should be attempted and checked with relatives whenever sub-nutrition or over-nutrition is suspected.

### Physical examination

Physical examination of an elderly patient is essentially the same as in a younger patient. One or two special points are worth noting in each system.

**General.** The general appearance in relation to age is often helpful. The youthful-looking old person usually has less underlying pathological change.

Cyanosis, malar flush, coldness of the extremities may indicate a low tissue oxygen saturation resulting from a low cardiac output.

An assessment of nutritional state and hydration should be noted, particularly when loss of weight or wasting are present. During the examination it is important to continue talking to the patient – it is reassuring and courteous and also often provides further invaluable or confirmatory history. Similarly, the patient's mood, appropriateness of response, etc. can all be assessed and recorded during physical examination.

**Cardiovascular system.** The apex beat is often difficult to feel, as are the pulses of the legs and feet; nevertheless, it is important to record the presence or absence of all peripheral pulses as well as the state of the arterial wall. It is often advantageous to examine the patient after exercise if that is the stimulus for symptoms.

**Respiratory system.** Age changes in the lungs themselves as well as weakness of the accessory muscles of respiration mean that physical signs may be less evident in the elderly. The most useful physical sign indicating lung disease is an increase in the respiratory rate, rising to 28/min or more. This sign may even precede radiological lung changes (Chapter 11).

**Central nervous system.** The fundi may be difficult to see and the pupils may require dilation; a good ophthalmoscope is needed and the doctor should be competent in its use. Ankle jerks are often absent, but this is not necessarily an indication of pathological change. Absent vibration sense in the legs is common and may not indicate disease. Where possible, the patient should be asked to stand so that his balance and gait can be assessed. Minor motor, co-ordination and sensory disturbances often only become apparent when this is done (Case 8).

**Endocrine.** Small goitres are often present and are easily missed. The testes are often smaller and harder than normal. Loss of hair is evident all over the body but is not associated with gross endocrine changes. Baldness is common and may be embarrassing to women.

**Alimentary system.** The dental state and whether or not false teeth are used should be recorded.

Physical signs in the acute abdomen in the elderly patient are often hard to elicit. The absence of bowel sounds may be the only indication that something is amiss.

**Locomotor system.** Abnormalities are common and often very important since they limit mobility. The state of the toenails should always be recorded. Opportunity should be taken to observe the patient getting out of a chair or bed and during walking – often this reveals that the locomotor problem is due to pain, weakness, stiffness or instability.

**Skin.** The state of the skin should be noted. A thin transparent skin on the back of the hands may indicate a similar state in the bones.

**Immune system.** Ageing is associated with a deterioration in the immediate and delayed response of the immune system to injury or infection. Practical implications of this are that the signs and symptoms of acute illness are often masked. In bronchopneumonia, for example, there often is no pyrexia, there is little change in the leucocyte count and the localising signs in the chest are minimal (*cf*. Chapter 11). It is also important in tuberculosis where an impaired immunological response may prevent a diagnostic response to the intradermal injection of tuberculin.

## The problem list

The use of problem-orientated medical records in the care of the elderly patient is invaluable and enables a continuing review of the individual's problems to be made. However, it must be stressed that building up the whole picture from a history and examination of the elderly patient takes time. It is probably best to start by listing the major presenting problem or problems and then adding to these as more information becomes available. Once the list has been made a plan of action can then be made for each of the problems on it. Initially, this may indicate the need for much more information which, in turn, may lead to the addition of further problems to the initial list.

## Further reading

Bromley D B (1974) *The Psychology of Human Ageing*. London: Penguin Books

Caird F I & Judge T G (1977) *Assessment of the Elderly Patient*. London: Pitman Medical

Hodkinson H M (1980) *Common Symptoms of Disease in the Elderly*. London: Blackwell

Weed L L (1971) *Medical Records, Medical Education and Patient Care*. Cleveland: Press of Case Western Research University

# CHAPTER 3

# Clinical Investigation in the Elderly

It is well recognised that the elderly suffer from more than one disease process at a time and that if a patient is to be treated correctly the diagnosis must be as precise as possible. One needs to know not only what is troubling the patient most, but what clinical problems may underlie his complaint and whether it is possible to put these right. Having talked to the patient, his relatives and others closest to him about his problems, and having examined him to assess mental and physical capacity we may now direct attention to the function of individual organs. This may involve chemical analysis of the blood, urine, faeces or sputum, and X-rays may be taken of bones, soft tissues and internal organs. Electrical tracings of heart or brain function, ultrasound recordings of the abdomen, computed tomography, and biopsies of skin, bone marrow or internal organs may also be necessary. The problems therefore, that face the clinical investigator are firstly, how much investigation is justified, secondly, how valuable are the tests and, thirdly, where should they be done?

**How much is investigation justified?** (Case 7)

This question can sometimes be very difficult to answer. The prime consideration must be the benefit which will accrue to the patient. It has already been pointed out that several disease processes commonly co-exist in the same patient and one of the commonest ways for illness to present in the elderly is 'failure to thrive'. In other words, the patient presents with symptoms of being unwell; further enquiry may only elicit a symptom such as tiredness or weakness, so that finding a cause is often difficult and time-consuming. Hence, it is often easier for the physician to ascribe the symptom to old age rather than to disease, or to give him a tablet in the hope that his symptom will go away. The treatment given will often depend on the physician's whim or whatever fashion is currently in vogue. Substances frequently prescribed are iron, vitamins, tranquillisers, anti-depressants, other types of 'happy' pills, anabolic steroids, 'cerebral activators' and other substances, sometimes classified under the heading of 'geripeutics'. The only beneficial effect of many of these is that of a placebo, while some will do more harm than good.

If the purpose of an investigation is explained, the elderly patient is usually most co-operative (Chapter 2: *the elderly patient as an individual*). It should, however, be remembered that the objective of any investigation should be to aid both the long- and short-term management plan of the individual in question. It should also be recognised that extensive investigation of multiple pathology is likely to cause considerable distress, discomfort and inconvenience. Objectives, therefore, should be clearly defined before embarking on a sequence of investigations.

Case 7 is a good example. A single blood sample revealed a general deficiency state which related to haemoglobin, potassium, calcium, magnesium, protein and iron while other blood tests suggested that vitamin D deficiency might also co-exist. The cause of the deficiencies could have been primary, ie. dietary, or secondary due to malabsorption. Other reasons such as blood loss from the gastrointestinal tract could have contributed. In view of this patient's great age one could perhaps have stopped investigations at this point and watched the effect of a good diet supplemented by vitamins, iron and other minerals. Such a policy would have had a relatively high chance of success but had it failed could have meant readmitting the patient to hospital. Since hospitals are potentially dangerous places for the old, further out-patient investigation could be justified, particularly as these investigations do not need to be unpleasant and distressing. Gastro-intestinal bleeding could be excluded by examination of the stools for occult blood, while simple skeletal X-ray, in fact, although not confirming vitamin D deficiency, revealed Paget's disease as a cause for one of the abnormal test results. Positive tests for blood in stools were further investigated by a barium examination of the upper gastrointestinal tract: this identified a treatable condition. As a result of these comparatively simple investigations it was possible to institute a simple medicinal régime which not only relieved the patient's symptoms but corrected the malabsorption. From the academic point of view it would have been interesting to have investigated her further by performing a small-bowel biopsy and in this way assess both the appearance and function of the small bowel more accurately. However, this did not seem justifiable since it is an unpleasant procedure with a potential risk which would not contribute to either the short-term or long-term management. Wherever possible, tests used to investigate elderly patients should be non-invasive. All should relate to the patient's health in terms of comfortable survival and it may be much better to obtain a specialist opinion before resorting to a battery of uncomfortable and potentially hazardous tests. For instance, it may be wiser to ask for the neuro-surgeon's opinion before deciding that a myelogram is necessary in a patient with paraplegia. Simple spinal X-rays may be sufficient to enable him to answer that an operation would be ineffective and an unpleasant procedure would be avoided.

## How valuable are the tests?

If one is to investigate an elderly person it is important to consider which tests are 'good value for money'. In other words, one wants to know which tests will give a high return in terms of treatable disease, or which tests may be valuable in indicating the need for further, more extensive investigation. It is almost universal that variation in individual parameters increases with increasing age. Whether this is due to 'physiological ageing' or latent disease is often unknown. Elucidation of this problem would allow the construction of much narrower 'normal ranges' in old age. This can only be achieved by a longitudinal or cohort study.

**Haematological tests** (Cases 3, 7).   Most of the standard haematological indices are unaffected by age so that the same values can be placed on these tests as in younger people. The incidence of anaemia, however, increases with age so that haematological investigation will tend to give a fairly high return in terms of treatable disease (Chapter 12).

The white cell count tends to fall with age and the range is usually given as from $3 \times 10^9 - 9 \times 10^9$/l.

The erythrocyte sedimentation rate (ESR) tends to rise with increasing age even in healthy individuals so that its value as a discriminator between health and disease is less in old age unless it is very high.

**Biochemical tests** (Case 7).   Many of the biochemical values which are accepted as normal in younger patients also apply to the elderly. These include the levels of sodium, potassium, chloride, bicarbonate, magnesium, phosphate, bilirubin and protein, as well as albumin and globulin. The ability of the kidney to excrete nitrogenous waste products in old age may be impaired so that the blood urea may be slightly elevated, a level of up to 10mmol/l being accepted as normal compared with a normal range of from 2.5 to 6.6 mmol/l (15–38 mg/100 ml) (Chapter 13: *renal function*): this is due to a reduced glomerular filtration rate. This observation is important because if the renal reserve is reduced the blood urea is likely to rise to even higher levels in situations of stress, so that patients with acute infection such as pneumonia might have blood urea levels of from 15–20 mmol/l (90–120 mg/100 ml). Such levels are usually indicative of renal failure in a younger patient but this does not often apply in the elderly. Similarly, the serum creatinine has a higher upper limit in old age, as does the serum uric acid. The diagnosis of renal failure is, therefore, more difficult and high uric acid levels do not always diagnose gout. Paradoxically, in the elderly it is not unusual to find patients with creatinine levels below 130 mmol/l who have an abnormally low creatinine clearance. This can probably be explained by a reduced rate of creatinine production secondary to a reduced lean body mass (Chapter 7).

High serum calcium concentrations are often found coincidentally in old people. More common causes for this include hyperparathyroidism, skeletal metastases, multiple myeloma and vitamin D intoxication. If no clinical symptoms are associated with hypercalcaemia due to hyper-parathyroidism, this is best left untreated (Chapter 7). Low levels of serum calcium may also be found in the elderly; this may indicate osteomalacia, a condition not uncommon in elderly housebound women living in northern climes (Chapter 7). Low calcium levels, however, may also be associated with low levels of albumin. Most laboratories use a simple formula which 'corrects' serum calcium concentration for albumin levels. This is particularly important in old age where ill health and sub-nutrition often lead to hypoalbuminaemia.

Low magnesium levels in the elderly may be more common than is generally realised and in one study one-third of the patients who attended a geriatric day hospital had low levels. Many of these had associated low calcium levels and the serum calcium level rose when magnesium was given in small doses by mouth. By far the commonest cause of mag-nesium deficiency was diuretic therapy. The deficiency also causes a hypokalaemia (low serum potassium) which is resistant to potassium replacement unless magnesium supplements are also given. Many old people have low serum potassium levels. While diuretic therapy is a fre-quent cause, deficient dietary intake of potassium is common. The serum potassium bears little relationship to total body stores; however, it remains a useful test in that it is the level of potassium in the plasma rather than that in cells which determines most of the symptoms. These include myocardial instability, muscle weakness, and gut atony.

**Endocrine tests.**   Because diabetes and disorders of the thyroid gland are common in old age, blood sugar estimations and tests of thyroid function may be of considerable value in diagnosing these conditions.

*Diabetes* (Chapter 13).   It is necessary to estimate the blood sugar level when this diagnosis is suspected. The problem that remains is the level of blood sugar that should be taken to indicate diabetes. It is probable that random levels of blood sugar of less than 8.3 mmol/l (150 mg/100 ml) are normal in elderly patients. Equally, levels over 11 mmol/l (198 mg/100 ml) are probably indicative of overt diabetes mellitus. The doubt arises in patients whose levels lie between 8.3 and 11 mmol/l. In these cases an oral glucose tolerance test may be necessary to determine the diagnosis. This means taking several blood samples. More simply, a fasting blood sugar of over 7.9 mmol/l (140 mg/100 ml) coupled with a blood sugar of over 11 mmol/l (198 mg/100 ml) 2 hours after taking 50 g of glucose orally is indicative of a diagnosis of overt diabetes mellitus. The normal accepted level of blood sugar 2 hours after taking 50 g of glucose by mouth is below 6.7 mmol/l (120 mg/100 ml) and many of the elderly have higher levels than this. Such people undoubtedly have carbohydrate intolerance if not diabetes mellitus, but treatment by dietary restrictions of carbohydrate is probably not justified and it is sufficient in the majority of these patients to warn them against the excessive consumption of carbohydrate.

Andres (1971) has constructed a nomogram as a guide to whether treatment is indicated (Fig. 3.1). Those patients with a blood sugar higher than the 5th percentile should probably be treated (Chapter 13).

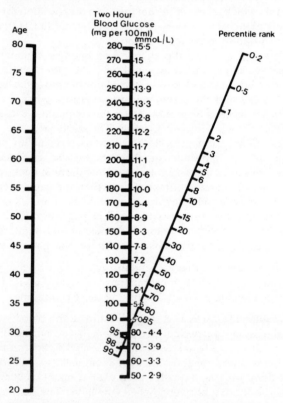

Figure 3.1   Nomogram relating glucose tolerance tests to age (Andres 1971)

*Thyroid disease.* The incidence of both overactivity and underactivity of the thyroid gland (Chapter 13) is of the order of from 1–2 per cent in patients admitted to geriatric units. Thyroid function tests may be of great value in distinguishing between the effects of ageing and hypothyroidism on mental function, and in highlighting hyperthyroidism as a cause of heart failure and pulse irregularity. In the case of hyper-thyroidism there is no doubt that an estimation of the serum triodothyronine ($T_3$) level is the most useful single test since the finding of a normal level undoubtedly excludes the condition. Similarly, a normal serum thyroid-stimulating-hormone (TSH) level will exclude the diagnosis of hypothyroidism. Old age alone may result in elevated TSH levels. The serum thyroxine ($T_4$) is a less specific test for either hypo-thyroidism or thyrotoxicosis, but it is easier to perform. Most laboratories now use the ratio of the $T_4$ to thyroid-binding globulin as a screening test for thyroid disease. If this is low, hypothyroidism is checked by measuring TSH, and if it is high, thyrotoxicosis is checked by estimating $T_3$. If doubts as to the diagnosis remains, the response of the pituitary and thyroid glands to an injection of thyrotrophin-releasing hormone (TRH) can be measured. This is particularly useful in the diagnosis of doubtful hyperthyroidism. In addition, it may also be useful in diagnosing doubtful cases of hypothyroidism where the basal TSH level is only minimally elevated, as patients with this condition show an exaggerated and prolonged TSH response to TRH.

**Radiological investigation.** Perhaps the two most valuable X-rays of the elderly patient are a PA chest and a straight X-ray of the abdomen taken to include both hip joints. Such X-rays not only give information on the state of the lungs, but by demonstrating much of the skeleton may be helpful in assessing the degree of osteoporosis or osteomalacia and demonstrating such disorders as Paget's disease and metastases from breast, lung and prostate. Further, the faecal content of the large bowel may be seen and this can be useful in the diagnosis of chronic constipation and high faecal impaction. Other changes including aortic and vascular calcification may also be seen (as well as gallstones and soft tissue shadows of kidney and bladder). More detailed X-rays of the elderly patient are probably of less value unless specifically indicated. Examples include X-ray examinations with barium meals and enemas to outline the upper and lower gastro-intestinal tract, and investigation of the urinary tract, with an intravenous pyelogram (IVP) in assessment of patients with urinary incontinence Chapter 14). Routine X-rays to show arthritis of the spine are of less value since this is nearly always present and often bears little relationship to the presence or absence of symptoms.

Ultrasonography is increasingly being used for the investigation of intra-abdominal lesions. Areas of particular value are in the identification of renal masses, liver secondaries and gallstones. The finding, however, can sometimes be misleading. Computed tomography of the brain, and even of the whole body, is now available in most advanced centres and can be particularly useful in providing accurate diagnoses in the elderly, and is particularly acceptable in that it is non-invasive. Nuclear magnetic resonance imaging (NMR) may be of even greater value in assessing the state of the elderly patient in that it may give a non-invasive estimate of tissue function. However, it is currently only available in some centres as a research tool and its value requires fuller assessment.

**Urinalysis.**   Urinalysis is probably less important in the elderly patient than it is in the young. Minor degrees of proteinuria are often found and may be relatively insignificant. Similarly, in diabetes, because the renal threshold of sugar is raised, glycosuria may not be present even when the blood sugar level is high (Chapter 13). On microscopy large numbers of pus cells usually indicate active infection. Haematuria, even microscopic, warrants investigation at any age.

**Bacteriological investigation.**   Bacteriological investigation of various body fluids can be of great value in the management and treatment of the elderly patient. It may, however, be difficult to get uncontaminated specimens of some fluids. Urine presents particular problems (Chapter 14). Nevertheless, bacteriological examination of sputum or pus from a joint effusion and other serous cavity may be a life-saving procedure by indicating the most effective antibiotic. Blood cultures themselves may be helpful in confirming the presence of an infective organism and its sensitivity to antibiotics and should be done whenever doubt exists in a pyrexial illness.

### Other investigations

All the usual investigations such as electroencephalography, electrocardiography, radio-isotope scanning, endoscopy and biopsies of bone, muscle, skin, artery and other tissues or organs may be of value in determining the management of appropriate patients.

Electrocardiographic tracings are frequently abnormal and community surveys have shown that about half of the elderly show some alteration in the wave form. Perhaps one of the most useful uses of the electrocardiograph is to determine digitalis sensitivity, which is often associated with low potassium levels (hypokalaemia). Twenty-four hour ambulatory cardiac monitoring, sometimes called the Dynamic Cardiograph (DCG) may be particularly useful in diagnosing cardiac arrhythmias, which may be associated with 'dizzy spells', falls, and other symptoms (Chapters 8 & 10).

Endoscopy, particularly gastroscopy and duodenoscopy, may be of great value in making definitive diagnoses. The elderly, surprisingly, seem to tolerate this type of examination extremely well and endoscopy may be preferable to a barium examination in some subjects. However, invasive investigations such as these should not be undertaken lightly. Endoscopy has developed recently to the stage that it can be used for the investigation and treatment of disorders of the pancreatic and common bile ducts. This is of great value in elderly patients unfit to withstand the stress of a laparotomy.

## Where should investigations be done?

Obviously many investigations in the elderly patient can be done on an out-patient basis. It is probably preferable to avoid admitting elderly patients to hospital for the purpose of investigation, unless sedation or an anaesthetic is necessary, because this will lessen the risk of infecting them with hospital organisms. It should, however, be borne in mind that many investigations are tiring for frail or elderly patients and consequently it may be necessary to provide day beds in which they can recover after their tests. If the geriatric day hospital is located within the DGH many patients would benefit by spending a day of investigation based in the day hospital. All investigations should be planned and discussed if full value is to be obtained from them and the elderly patient inconvenienced as little as possible.

It must be remembered that the main purpose of investigation is to initiate treatment that will make the patient more comfortable and improve the quality of his life. Specialists in other disciplines may have different priorities and have difficulty in understanding the need for investigation (or for that matter the treatment) without prior consultation and explanation. Consultation with other specialists concerned with investigation, although often forgotten, should always be obligatory. Only by such interdisciplinary consultation and co-operation will it be possible for those practising geriatric medicine to become practically acquainted with senile pathology and surmount its difficulties.

## Further reading

Andres R (1971) Ageing and diabetes, *Med Clin N Am*, **55**, 835–846

Editorial (1982) The ESR – an outdated test? *Lancet*, **1**, 377

Hodkinson H M (1977) *Biochemical Diagnosis of the Elderly*. London: Chapman & Hall

Sowell J M, Spooner L L R, Dixon A K & Rubenstein D (1981) Screening investigations in the elderly. *Age & Ageing*, **10**, 165–168

CHAPTER 4

# Social Problems and the Elderly

## Introduction

Patients are often referred by other hospital departments to the geriatric department as a 'social problem'. Similarly, general practitioners refer patients to the social services department because they present a 'social problem'. In both cases the request is either for advice concerning continuing management of the 'social problem' or for 'disposal', as though the individual were a piece of refuse. The importance of multidisciplinary consultation in the care and management of the ill elderly person has already been stressed (Chapter 1: *ascertainment*). If an organisation exists whereby such consultation is easy to achieve, the prevention of social stress and thereby a 'social problem' then becomes easier.

*Definition:* 'A social problem may be defined as arising when the continuing existence of an individual in the community causes social stress which is perceived to be unacceptable to those concerned with that individual and for the individual himself.'

## The causes of social problems

Social stress sufficient to cause a social problem may arise for several reasons which may be listed in the following ways.

**Physical disability** (Cases 2, 5, 7). This is one of the commonest underlying causes. It is easy to understand why this should be, since disability, whether due to age or disease, sufficient to prevent an individual performing the normal everyday activities of daily living means that he needs someone's help. If there is no one to help he will suffer from neglect in some way. How the neglect effects the individual varies, but it inevitably increases both his physical incapacity and his social incompetence so that sooner or later a cry for help will be made either by the individual himself or by someone who is connected with him or knows about him. Often this type of physical disability is attributed to 'just old age', which is discussed in Chapter 6, while other causes are discussed in other chapters, eg. 7 and 8.

**Mental disability** (Case 6).   This again is a very common cause of a social problem. It can result either from acute or chronic brain failure or an affective mental disorder such as depressive illness. These problems are discussed in greater detail in Chapters 6 and 9 (Cases 8 and 9).

**Social incompetence.**   While this can arise as a result of both physical and mental malfunction, there are a few people who are just bad managers and always have been. In early life they are often supported by relatives or friends, but as they grow older either their relatives or lifetime associates die or desert them, so that they are left alone. In these cases physical and mental aspects may play no part and support has to be provided by the social services department. Such people are uncommon in geriatric practice and before labelling an elderly individual socially incompetent the clinician must be sure there is no underlying physical or mental impairment. (Case 8).

**Difficult personalities** (Cases 3 and 5).   It is often said that as a person ages he becomes a caricature of his previous personality. People with abnormal personalities may well give rise to social stress which results as referral as a social problem. These range from the strong-willed, dominant person who will often accept neglect and discomfort as a reasonable price to pay for independence, through the chronic manipulator whose skill in using frailties, situations and human beings to his own advantage will sometimes drive relatives to suicide, to the frankly abnormal who may lead the life of a recluse or present with 'Diogenes' syndrome', collecting large amounts of useless material such as newspapers, and living in dirt and squalor.

**Antisocial behaviour** (Cases 2, 3, 4 and 8)

This may take many forms from aggressive, noisy behaviour to dirty habits such as the faecal smearing of walls or hiding 'parcels' of excreta in drawers or cupboards. Studies have shown that the most difficult problem for carers to overcome is lack of sleep. Some elderly parents may have inverted sleep rhythms, so that they sleep all day and are awake and noisy at night. Relief for these carers as well as others confronted with social problems is urgently needed if long-term care is to be avoided.

**Attitudes in relation to social problems** (Cases 1, 3, 5, 6, 7)

**The social worker.**   One of the major functions of the social worker is to discover the wishes of the elderly client, assess how realistic these are and, after discussion with the client and others, organise appropriate support to enable the client to achieve his wish. Opposition to the client's wish may come from relatives, friends, neighbours and health professionals and it is part of the social worker's task to assess these objections and allay fears, so that the wishes of the elderly client, if reasonable, may be fulfilled. The social worker's problem is to decide what is reasonable, and this can only be achieved if her attitude is that of friend and arbiter to the elderly client. A social worker must, as far as is humanly possible, see that the wishes of the client are carried out. Sometimes these may seem unrealistic and impracticable; nevertheless, if sufficiently motivated, some people can overcome great disability and handicap and continue to live in their own homes despite the opposition of relatives, friends and neighbours, and health care professionals.

It is not uncommon, when such strong-willed people refuse to do what others would wish of them and insist on their human rights, that the judgement of the social worker may be called into question by the relatives and others. In these circumstances the social worker's rôle is often unenviable. Nevertheless, if the wishes of the elderly client are to be fulfilled it is vital that the social worker displays tact and patience while allowing the relatives and others to work through their fears and anxieties.

**Health professionals.** Doctors, nurses and other health professionals have varying attitudes towards the 'social problem'. In some cases patients are called social problems because the doctor cannot see a solution to the medical problem. Since he is unwilling to admit the failure of his medical skill he blames the social circumstances for the failure to discharge the patient from his hospital bed. Similarly, the social stress imposed on relatives by their physically and mentally handicapped elderly dependents in their homes may pressure the family doctor to ignore the physical or mental problem and describe the patient as a social problem. Careful multi-disciplinary assessment of the individual's physical, mental and social state is essential before any such decision is made, and the individual's own wishes must be taken into account. (Chapter 5)

Elderly patients often acquire the label 'social problem' in a casualty department. Thus, a little old lady living alone, subject to frequent falls, is 'sent in' by neighbours using the emergency ambulance late on a Friday evening. As the patient cannot be sent home she is admitted reluctantly as a 'social admission'. Unfortunately, the label may direct the hospital doctors into finding a social solution to the neglect of the patient's actual problem – eg. recurrent falls. An identical younger patient would have had EEG, CT brain scan, 24-hour ECG, blood sugar series, and so on, before any mention of a social solution. The point is that relief of the underlying medical problem invariably cures the 'social problem'.

**Relatives, friends and neighbours.** It is very easy to understand the anxieties and pressures which can be placed upon relatives, friends and neighbours of an elderly person who is becoming socially incompetent. They are often afraid that harm will befall them so that relatives will claim they cannot be left alone. 'What happens if he/she falls?' is the question asked. Some of these problems can be seen in Case 1 and some solutions are suggested. While it is of little comfort, it is important to realise that living is a very dangerous business. It is much safer to be dead. In other words, every age has its hazards and risks, the problem is how to decide which risks are acceptable and which are not. Finally, the individual's own wishes may be such that the risk will have to be ignored or accepted.

It is important to remember that elderly dependent people may be eligible for an attendance allowance. Further, close relatives who spend at least 35 hours per week caring for a severely disabled elderly person may be eligible for an invalid care allowance, but only one of these allowances will usually be payable. Finally, if it is considered that the individual represents a public health hazard or is in such a state as to be unable to care for himself, the case may be brought to the notice of a magistrate who on the advice of two doctors may order admission to hospital for a period of 21 days, under Section 47 of the Public Assistance Act.

**The general public.** It is beyond the scope of this handbook to look at social policy and legislation and the attitude of the general public, who are often too busy living their own lives to be much concerned with the care of the elderly unless they themselves are personally involved with an elderly dependent. When disasters occur, such as an elderly person dying from hypothermia (Chapter 13), or being found six months after death, there is usually a public outcry of horrified concern. As the number of elderly in advanced societies increases, the importance of the group as a political entity becomes apparent. Politicians of all parties have to recognise that the needs of the elderly are diverse and that in addition to medical care, special consideration must be given to pensions, housing and both leisure and cultural activities. Indeed, it is slowly becoming recognised that the rising tide of sick old people in advanced societies threatens to impose intolerable strains on financial and manpower resources. The problem is becoming so great that it can probably only be solved by a preventive approach. Priority must be given to preserving community life, particularly family structures, human relationships and social groups with community sense. Retirement must not be allowed to become an eventless interregnum between work and death but should be recognised as an opportunity for individuals to make an increased contribution to society. Society should have views on this, but before it can have such views it must be educated.

## Pre-retirement education

Most people who retire between the ages of 60 and 65 will have another 15 to 20 years of life ahead of them. If retirement is to be enjoyed then it should be planned. The basic requirements for a happy retirement are money and good health, which if present will enable the individual to engage in recreational and leisure pursuits.

Education about the ageing process and the problems of life after retirement should form part of all educational programmes. It is probably never too early to start and certainly some form of education concerning ageing and the ageing process should be undertaken prior to leaving school. Advice on pensions and savings needs to be given early in life. At present, many elderly people find, as a result of inflation, that they cannot manage on savings and social security pensions and have to go out to work to supplement their incomes. It may well be that society could reserve for the elderly certain types of work particularly suited to their aptitudes. Obviously, with a high level of unemployment, this is very difficult to organise.

## Pre-retirement and post-retirement courses

In many parts of the world, and in the United Kingdom in particular, both pre- and post-retirement courses are being run by local adult education departments. These may take the form of residential week-end courses, day release courses or evening courses; they focus on the various problems which the individual is liable to face in retirement, and provide advice on financial matters, on health, on leisure and recreation and on the use of the social services. It is generally agreed that the most successful pre-retirement course is relatively small, having between twelve and twenty students. This enables the tutor and lecturers to conduct seminars and get to know individual members of the course. These small groups interact well and individuals find they are more interesting. Lecturers to both pre-retirement and post-retirement courses need careful briefing. The Pre-retirement Association has appropriate lecture notes available and these should be studied. It is most important that lecturers should concentrate on the positive aspects of retirement and on the gain and fulfillment that can be achieved during retirement. The more negative and depressing aspects such as ill-health and bereavement, poverty and loneliness must be faced in a positive manner, and ways of recognising and mitigating them suggested.

## Community services (Case 6)

The vast majority of the elderly wish to remain in their own homes. In order to enable them to do this it is important that good community services should exist, and be available to the community health team. The community health team usually comprises a general practitioner with a supporting health visitor and a nurse. The attachment of nursing personnel to individual general practices ensures that greater cover of the elderly clientele can be achieved. Nurses and health visitors can develop continuing relationships with patients and their families in conjunction with their general practitioner. While the rôle of the nurse and doctor is primarily concerned with the treatment of ill-health, the health visitor is concerned with the prevention of ill-health and its consequences, as well as its early detection, and the surveillance of high-risk groups such as the recently bereaved or the recently discharged from hospital. She is also responsible for a certain amount of health education, the identification of needs and the mobilisation of appropriate resources.

The resources available to the health visitor should include those of luncheon clubs, day centres, equipment, housing modifications, home helps, meals-on-wheels, laundry support and voluntary visiting. Most hospital geriatric services and local authority services for the elderly run holiday relief schemes to enable caring relatives to take a holiday. Accommodation should be booked well in advance of the proposed holiday period so that the most suitable place may be found for the person concerned.

## Voluntary Services

Many Voluntary Services play an important part in helping to solve and prevent social problems. The most prominent of these is Age Concern which has local committees in most towns. It publishes an excellent booklet yearly, Your Rights, which lists all services available to the elderly. Voluntary Organisations are also responsible for the initiation of many schemes which help the elderly to remain in their own homes: examples are the Association of Carers, Care Attendant Schemes, and 'Sitting in' Services.

## Specialist housing for the elderly (Case 1)

All local authority distric housing services reserve a certain proportion of ordinary council housing for the elderly. In addition, most housing departments have developed special housing schemes for the elderly, known as Category 2 housing, whereby flatlets and maisonettes are supervised by trained wardens. Similarly, voluntary organisations have established housing associations with specialist housing and accommodation.

It has been disappointing to note that tenants in such property are not maintained longer in the community than those in conventional housing. A reappraisal of the rôle and operation of sheltered housing is badly needed. It is possible that the provision of more staff to supervise residents in sheltered housing may enable them to remain there longer. Some experimental schemes have been initiated (sometimes called Category 2½ or Part 2½ accommodation) and early analysis seems promising.

All such special category housing is linked to the Warden by an *alarm system*. Modern communication systems suggest that an extension of alarm systems, via telephone or radio links, may provide a simple way of establishing a link between the elderly and their carers. Little research has been done to establish the value of such 'alarm systems' and it is possible that these systems may be overvalued and expensive.

It is important therefore before installing such a system, to weigh its cost/effectiveness against the employment of additional warden cover.

## Residential accommodation (Cases 1, 2, 7)

A small number of old people cannot survive in the community even in sheltered accommodation and require the hotel type of residential accommodation which is provided by the local authority social services department. The recommended provision is twenty-five places per 1,000 elderly and includes accommodation for the mentally frail as well as the physically handicapped elderly. This accommodation is quite often purpose-built and is staffed by a resident officer in charge with some supporting staff. The frailty of residents in this accommodation is, however, increasing and it seems likely that staff provision will also have to increase so that the appropriate level of care may be provided.

In addition to this statutory accommodation a considerable number of places is available in private nursing homes and rest homes. Local authorities and local health authorities ensure standards by licensing, respectively, rest homes and nursing homes.

Recent legislation on social security supplementation for clients on low incomes requiring such accommodation has opened it up to a much wider section of the population. As a result, in some areas, there has been such an expansion of rest home places in the private sector that they now outnumber those in the public sector.

## Long-term hospital care

An individual may develop such severe mental or physical handicap that his care places intolerable stress on those looking after him at home or in residential accommodation. He should then be admitted to a hospital unit especially designed for the longer-stay patient. This particular category of care has been long neglected, for there is little more to be done for these patients from the curative medical standpoint, even though they can live lives of considerable quality if they are given the chance by being adequately supported by health professionals and others. In this type of unit the accent needs to be placed more on leisure activities than on traditional hospital care (Chapter 9). It is important also to try to give creative rôles to patients even though they may be severely handicapped. If this can be achieved the individual can retain his self respect and feel that he still has a useful part to play in life. A considerable social work rôle remains to be explored in this particular field.

A perennial problem of long-term care is whether people with mental impairment should be mixed with those who are physically incapacitated but mentally normal. One of the stigmas of the long-stay hospital is that the patients are 'geriatric', an adjective which is beginning to have derisive connotations in various circumstances both in television programmes and in the House of Commons. There is no doubt that it stems from the fact that many patients in long-stay units have brain damage and consequently impaired mental performance; this is usually coupled with physical incapacity so that the patient is immobile. Under these circumstances a patient is normally accepted in a medical long-stay unit where about three-quarters of the other patients will be like him. If, however, the patient is mobile and therefore liable to wander or has other unacceptable behaviour he should then be cared for in a psychiatric long-stay unit. In either case the unit should be so organised to help individuals to achieve their maximum potential.

## Further reading

Brearley C P (1975) *Social Work, Ageing and Society*. London: Routledge & Kegan Paul

Brearley C P (1977) *Residential Work with the Elderly*. London: Routledge & Kegan Paul

Bromley D B (ed) (1984) *Gerontology – Social and Behavioural Perspectives*. London: Croom Helm

Butler A, Oldman C & Greve J (1983) *Sheltered Housing for the Elderly. Policy, Practice and Consumer*. George Allen & Unwin

Goffman E (1971) *Asylums*. London: Penguin (Pelican) Books

Gray M & Wilcock G (1981) *Our Elders*. Oxford University Press

Hanley, I & Hodge, J (eds) (1984) *Psychological Approaches to the Care of the Elderly*. London: Croom Helm.

Hobman D (1978) *The Social Challenge of Ageing*. London: Croom Helm

MacLennan W J, Grant J, Forbes B, Urquhart J M & Taylor-Brown O (1983) The relevance of health to rehousing in old age. *Health Bulletin*, **41**, 181–187

Taylor, R & Gilmore, A (1982) *Current Trends in British Gerontology*. London: Gower.

# CHAPTER 5

# Treatment and Management of the Elderly Patient

## Introduction

The first four chapters of this book have stressed the importance of accurate assessment of the elderly patient. This not only means clinical investigation and diagnosis but also the physical, mental and social assessment of the individual's capacity which is essential in the effective planning of treatment and management.

Since the elderly are often frail and severely disabled, it is most important to set therapeutic goals which are attainable. Expecting too much may engender a sense of failure which will negate any further attempts at rehabilitation. The goals set must be clearly defined and understood by all members of the therapeutic team and the patient and his relatives so that the response of the elderly patient to treatment can be accurately monitored and appropriate adjustments made at regular intervals. The reviews are best made at a multi-disciplinary case conference involving as many members of the therapeutic team as are necessary.

## The case conference (Case 3)

Elderly patients referred to the hospital geriatric service may be treated as out-patients, day-patients or in-patients. Out-patients are usually referred by a general practitioner for an opinion on a clinical or clinico-social condition. The consultant will see the patient at an out-patient department and collate information supplied to him by the general practitioner, the patient himself, a relative or a friend, and perhaps a social worker. He may then be able to suggest a solution to the problem raised by the general practitioner. However, providing an answer may require the performance of various special investigations on the patient as an out-patient or, if this is not practicable, assessment may require admission to hospital or a day hospital. Recently discharged patients may also be followed up for a limited time, as out-patients, in order to monitor progress and ensure that the therapeutic goals already set are being achieved and maintained.

At the end of each of the case histories (pp. 1–25) a problem list has been constructed to show some of the possible effects that could result from the medical problems. Various actions which can be taken to counteract these effects are given in the third column of the problem list. These lists are not intended to be comprehensive and the discerning, imaginative reader may well be able to add to the number of possible effects and, therefore, the possible actions it may be necessary to take.

A case conference is rarely practicable or, indeed, desirable in a busy out-patient clinic. However, for the in-patient or the day-patient a case conference is vital if adequate treatment and management plans are to be made (Fig. 5.1). The problem lists illustrate (as can be seen from the keys) that different health care professionals may be involved in treatment and management. We also have to involve the patient himself and his relatives. Friends, neighbours and voluntary workers may also be concerned and able to play a part in providing appropriate social contacts through day centres, luncheon clubs or visiting schemes.

With so many people likely to be involved in the treatment and management of a single patient it can easily be seen that chaos will arise unless their actions are carefully co-ordinated and understood. Hence, the

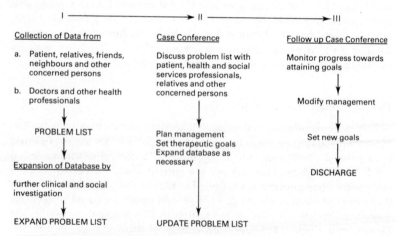

Figure 5.1   Flow diagram to illustrate the place of the case conference

need for a case conference where details can be discussed and the varying assessments of the health care professionals stated. The doctor, as leader of the team, can then agree with his colleagues the rôle each will play in

Table 5.1   Case Conference Check List

Medical problems: *diagnosis and treatment*
Social state and interaction with medical state
Special problems: *hearing*
          *speech*
          *vision*
Mental state: *confused*
        *depressed*
        *alert*
Urinary control
Bowel function
Teeth

| Physical capacity: | *feeding* | *dressing* |
| | *sitting in bed/chair* | *toileting* |
| | *transferring bed/chair* | *bathing* |
| | *standing* | *household tasks* |
| | *walking: with help* | *cooking ability* |
| | *with aid* | *shopping* |
| | *alone* | |

Set goals for attainment
Information to be discussed with patient and relatives

relation to the patient, decide the priorities and set the therapeutic goals. These, for the sake of clarity, should be described in simple 'performance' terms, eg. standing unsupported, walking with a stick, etc. As will be seen from the problem lists, elderly patients have many problems, some of which they recognise and many which they do not. Problems which may seem of prime importance to the therapeutic team may be relatively unimportant to the individual, whereas a relatively simple overlooked problem, such as a corn or the inability to perform some specific task, may cause the patient the greatest hardship. In deciding priorities for treatment the wishes and views of the patient must be sought since the major objective of all treatment is to improve the quality of his life. The more rapidly this can be done the better it is for the individual. A check list similar to that shown in Table 5.1 will help to ensure that information is complete.

It is beyond the scope of this handbook to discuss the rights of patients and ethical problems, but it must be stressed that the rights of the individual must always be borne in mind and his wishes respected. It is important to remember that the elderly frequently have great difficulty in making up their minds and often the more information they are given the more difficult it becomes. Explanations, therefore, must be simple, and plenty of time must be allowed for discussion of the pros and cons.

The case conference, although time-consuming, is essential if the best overall results are to be achieved for it provides a good forum in which to discuss ethical problems and propound varying views concerning correct patient care. As such it is a most useful teaching and training ground for medical, nursing and social work students as well as providing a base for the continuing audit of progress.

## Drug therapy

While drugs play a very important part in the management of many medical problems, drug therapy itself is not without its drawbacks in the elderly. In recent years a considerable amount of work has been done on the effect ageing has on the way in which drugs are absorbed, distributed, metabolised and excreted (pharmacokinetics), and on the effects drugs have on target organs (pharmacodynamics). When one considers the alterations which occur in various physiological systems with ageing it is hardly surprising that pharmacological preparations may have different effects on older people than they do on the young, and may be absorbed, metabolised and excreted in different ways and at different rates. It is important, therefore, when prescribing to remember some basic general principles in relation to the use of drugs.

## Basic principles

1 *All drugs should be considered potentially harmful to the elderly patient.* Drugs are given to relieve symptoms and consequently, before a drug is prescribed, the symptom must be viewed in relation to the distress it is causing, and the adverse effects of the drug to be used must be weighed against the distress caused by the symptom.

Ankle swelling is a good example, as it is a relatively common occurrence in old age and has many causes. Diuretics are commonly prescribed to relieve the symptom, often without reference to the cause, and adverse reactions such as urinary incontinence, a fall in blood pressure after standing or taking exercise (Chapter 10: *postural hypotension*) or potassium depletion with associated weakness and lethargy, may occur. If the ankle swelling is related to heart failure then almost certainly the diuretic was correctly prescribed. However, ankle swelling is often due to immobility and is then better treated by elevating the legs or using elastic stockings and/or elastic bandages. In these patients a diuretic is ineffective and its use quite unjustified.

Having decided that a drug is necessary it is essential to monitor the effect of that drug to ensure that it is doing its job and not causing any ill effects. Equally, it is important to confirm that the drug has indeed achieved the initial therapeutic objective – if not it should be reviewed, stopped or changed. The patient's compliance should also be confirmed. It is important to remember that higher blood concentrations per dose may result from altered metabolism and diminished excretion so that a lower or less frequent dose of the drug may be needed.

2 *When giving a drug treat the patient as an individual and titrate the dose of the drug in relation to the patient's response.* The use of L-dopa in the treatment of Parkinson's disease (Chapter 8) is a good example of this principle. The elderly patient will often suffer adverse effects from L-dopa if the dose given is too large or the increment is made too quickly, and initial doses may be so small that in younger patients they would seem homeopathic.

3 *Large loading doses are very rarely necessary unless a rapid response is needed.* For instance, the normal loading dose of digitalis needed in the younger patient will be as effective in the older patient. However, the dose necessary to maintain therapeutic response may be as low as 62.5 $\mu$g and rarely exceeds 250 $\mu$g, the response to a particular dose being dependent upon both body build and renal function.

4 *Drug régimes must be kept constantly under review.* Since the elderly suffer from multiple pathology it may frequently be necessary to use more than one drug in a patient, and the possibility of interaction between one drug and another must always be borne in mind.

5 *Routine repeat prescriptions should never be given to elderly patients for longer than a period of about three months.* For example, it has been shown that maintenance digitalis therapy is unnecessary in about 70 per cent of people receiving it. Diuretics also can eventually be discontinued without adverse effects.

6 *Keep drug régimes simple.* The elderly have difficulty in managing complex drug régimes and only three or four different preparations can be given successfully at one time to the majority of patients. Complex régimes also greatly increase the incidence of drug side effects and interactions. It is, therefore, unwise to prescribe more than this number of drugs if self-administration is to be relied upon. Fortunately for the elderly, omission of medication is the most frequent error. If this were not so the incidence of symptoms due to the ill effects of drugs (iatrogenic disease) might be considerably higher.

### Absorption, metabolism and excretion of drugs

In prescribing drugs for elderly patients it is important to bear in mind some of the changes which occur in their absorption, metabolism and excretion. Adverse drug reactions are very common in old people and can occur either as a result of the patient being given too large a dose or by altered pharmacological handling resulting in higher drug levels and a prolonged drug life.

## Absorption

Ageing has very little effect on drug absorption. Indeed changes in liver function mean that less of the drug is removed as it passes from the portal system through the liver. This means that many drugs, including propranolol, achieve higher initial plasma levels in the elderly. Moreover gastro-intestinal motility may be altered, as a result of ageing changes in the gut, or due to the effect of other drugs (eg. anticholinergics, laxatives) so that drug levels may be affected and peak levels may take longer to achieve.

## Metabolism

Age-related changes in enzymes involved in oxidative metabolism, mean that it takes longer for the body to eliminate drugs mainly metabolised by this route. There is less problem with agents eliminated by conjugation in the liver, since this process does not change with age.

## Protein binding

A low serum albumin concentration means that less protein is available for binding a drug so that the proportion of free and, consequently, active drug is increased. Ageing itself causes a fall in the serum albumin concentration, but the process is often exacerbated by disease and subnutrition. A reduction of binding sites on the albumin molecule may also occur with ageing, thereby also increasing free (active) drug levels.

**Excretion.**    Diminished renal excretion undoubtedly plays a large part in the retention of some drugs in the elderly (Chapter 13). The formulation of most drugs as weak bases may also be a factor in their defective elimination. It is well known that basic drugs are better reabsorbed by the kidney if the urine is alkaline. Many elderly subjects live on reduced incomes and have low protein intakes, with the result that their urine tends to be alkaline. Further, old people often drink less fluid and consequently pass less urine. Both these factors will lead to higher blood drug concentrations. Finally, reduced protein intake may also lead to low plasma albumin levels which in turn may lead to less effective protein binding of drugs so that more free drug is available to produce an effect.

**Rehabilitation and the Adjustment of the environment** (Cases 1, 2, 3, 5)
(Chapter 4)

While drugs can be used to control the individual's internal environment
his ability to perform the ordinary acts of daily living are probably of even
greater importance to him, and while doctors and nurses have an important part to play in the adjustment of an individual's internal environment, the remedial therapists have an equally important rôle to play in the
adjustment of the individual's external environment. By active educative
exercises, the physiotherapist can increase the range of joint and limb
movement and thereby the general mobility of the patient. Mobility may
also be increased by the use of various walking aids, while patients who
are unable to walk may be capable of being taught to lead independent
lives in wheelchairs. Obviously the individual may also be limited in his
ability to overcome obstacles such as steps and stairs which may exist in
his home. It is important for the physiotherapist to visit the home to make
a first-hand assessment of the obstacles which may interfere with the
patient's discharge. Close liaison with the primary medical care team and
the social worker concerned is also important.

Similarly, the occupational therapist has a vital rôle to play in training
the individual to perform the ordinary normal activities of daily living.
With the physiotherapist, the occupational therapist needs to ensure that
the patient can get out of bed, get dressed, walk to the lavatory, use it,
walk back to bed, can get undressed and get into bed. If the individual
can perform all these functions unaided then he should be able to leave
hospital and live at home. Such skills as cooking, housekeeping and
shopping are luxuries which, however desirable, should not prevent discharge, since home support in the form of meals-on-wheels, home help
and the laundry service can be provided through the social services
department. Nevertheless, it has to be accepted that frail, disabled elderly
people who have recently been in hospital are likely to have many accidents at home. Falls can occur as the result of unsteadiness, and some
simple precautions should be taken to mitigate these if they do occur.
Patients should be actively taught how to pick themselves up off the floor.
If this cannot be achieved appropriate alarm systems should be devised
and blankets kept within reach of the floor so that the patient can keep
warm if he has to remain on the floor overnight or until help arrives.

The amount of time that a physiotherapist or occupational therapist can
spend on an individual patient is extremely limited, and it is thus essential that the nurse should take an active part in the rehabilitation process.
Examples include encouraging the patient to dress rather than be dressed;
getting him to go to the lavatory rather than use a commode; and ensuring
that he spends as much time as possible practising walking. In the

geriatric setting, the nurse in addition to fulfilling her traditional rôles should consider herself to be a 'nurse therapist' and a full member of the rehabilitation team (Chapter 8).

## Anaesthesia and surgery

Many doctors other than the geriatrician are likely to be involved in the care of the elderly patient. Some surgeons have many elderly patients and this particularly applies in such surgical specialities as orthopaedics, urology and ophthalmology. It is important to remember that age is almost never a bar to surgery.

Equally, the modern anaesthetist is so skilled that there is hardly an elderly patient who cannot have an anaesthetic. The basic principles of the treatment and management of illness which have been outlined in this chapter should be borne in mind when elderly patients need to have an anaesthetic and be treated surgically. Close co-operation between the surgical/anaesthetic team and the geriatric medical team should be encouraged. Early mobilisation with adequate pain relief and specialist measures to avoid the development of bed sores can do much to speed recovery and shorten the hospital stay. The organisation of joint clinical areas between either orthopaedic or urological surgeons and geriatricians has been shown to be an effective way of improving patient management in some areas.

## Bed sores

A bed sore is essentially the result of prolonged pressure cutting off the blood supply to an area of skin and sub-cutaneous tissue. This situation arises where illness immobilises a patient or alters skin sensation. Damage is particularly likely to occur where tissue viability is further impaired by chronic illness, sub-nutrition or urinary incontinence.

The problem should be tackled by identifying patients at particular risk and then instituting preventive measures. The most important of these is changing the position of the patient at least every two hours so that no area of the skin is subjected to prolonged ischaemia. Attention should also be given to the patient's position in a bed or chair. If this is not done, horizontal movement may cause shearing of a blood vessel connecting deep and sub-cutaneous tissues. Various lotions and creams such as zinc cream (Phisohex) are of value in preventing sores. Their mode of action is obscure but may include antiseptic, nutritional, greasing and moisturising effects. Attention to the general condition of the patient, such as correcting anaemia, avoiding dehydration or replacing vitamins, is yet another important ancillary measure. Various cushions and mattresses have been devised to redistribute skin pressure, including large air-cell intermittent pressure mattresses, cushions or mattresses containing polystyrene balls and synthetic gel cushions. It must be emphasised that these are merely aids to nursing and are no substitute for regularly changing the position of a patient. It must also be remembered that pressure sores may have their origin outside the ward, in the operating theatre, in the ambulance, on the 'casualty trolley', or on the X-ray table. Appropriate mattresses/cushions need to be provided in these areas.

Once pressure areas have developed the treatments are legion. Every nursing sister has her own favourite concoction. The general principles are to control sepsis and to remove dead tissue so that granulation tissue can form and the sore heal by epithelialisation. Infection can be controlled by antiseptics, eg. cetrimide. Powerful antiseptics should be avoided because these will kill regenerating epithelium. Dead tissue (eschar) should be removed by cutting with scissors until either bleeding occurs or the patient complains of pain. Care should, of course, be taken to avoid further pressure on the sore. Where the problem is particularly intractable resort may have to be made to flotation or low-pressure air bed. Reconstructive plastic surgery may be of great value in selected cases.

### Further reading

Anderson W F, Caird F I, Kennedy R D & Schwartz D (1982) *Gerontology and Geriatric Nursing*. Sevenoaks: Hodder & Stoughton

Barton A & Barton M (1981) *The Management and Prevention of Pressure Sores*. London: Faber & Faber

Brocklehurst J C & Tucker J S (1980) *Progress in Geriatric Day Care*. King Edward's Hospital Fund for London.

Brocklehurst J C (ed) (1984) *Geriatric Pharmacology and Therapeutics*. Oxford: Blackwell

Caird F I, Kennedy R D & Williams B O (1983) *Practical Rehabilitation of the Elderly*. London: Pitman

Crooks J & Stevenson I H (eds) (1979) *Drugs and the Elderly: Perspectives in Geriatric Clinical Pharmacology*. London: MacMillan

Denham M J (1980) *Treatment of Medical Problems in the Elderly*. Lancaster: MTP

Denham M J (1983) *Care of the Long Stay Elderly Patient*. London: Croom Helm

MacDonald E T & MacDonald J B (1982) *Drug Treatment in the Elderly*. Chichester: Wiley

MacLennan W J, Shepherd A N & Stevenson I H (1984) *The Elderly*. Berlin: Springer-Verlag

# CHAPTER 6

# It's Just Old Age

Although ageing is associated with some decline in organ and tissue function, most of the symptoms and disabilities afflicting old people result from disease. Most laymen and all too many professionals, however, consider that failing faculties, severe disability and multiple aches and pains are inevitable and irreversible concomitants of ageing. A 40-year-old man who experiences chest pain requests an urgent home visit from his doctor. If an 85-year-old woman experiences the same symptom she is likely to shrug her shoulders and say: 'What can you expect? It's just old age'. It is vital that the general public and professionals should be educated in the differences between the effects of ageing and those of disease. Failure to appreciate these can have disastrous consequences both for individuals and for the heavily-stretched supporting services.

## Hearing

Deafness is a common but not inevitable accompaniment of ageing. It is partly due to the natural death of irreplaceable neurones in the acoustic nerve. Environment may also be of major importance. At the one extreme is the Russian peasant who at the age of 90 can hear a pin drop; conversely, there is the Clydeside boiler maker who may be severely deaf in early middle age.

Although their hearing is impaired for all frequencies of sound, old people have most difficulty in picking up high-pitched sounds. This means that, even if a hearing aid is used, sounds may be badly distorted.

In the cochlea the receptors for soft sounds are more severely degenerated than those for loud ones, which may account for a normal voice being inaudible, but shouting being painful – a phenomenon known as 'recruitment'. The reasonable request 'Please speak up, I'm hard of hearing' may be followed by the irate complaint 'There's no need to shout. I'm not deaf'. Slow, well-articulated speech with the speaker's facial movements clearly visible to the patient is the answer to this problem.

The patient may also have difficulty in focusing onto sounds. This manifests itself at social gatherings where he has difficulty in separating the conversation of his neighbour from the general background noise. It may also account for the state of confusion which the hoot of a horn induces in an elderly person crossing the road.

The frequency of deafness due to ageing (presbyacusis) should not lead to the neglect of other possible causes of deafness in old age. Old people were brought up in a pre-antibiotic era when middle ear infections were extremely common. At a more mundane level many elderly people suffer from deafness, dizziness and buzzing in their ears simply because their ears are stuffed with wax.

The diagnosis of presbyacusis is made from the configuration of the pure tone audiogram, as in many cases, the loss of hearing may be greater in one ear. Speech frequency varies between 500 and 20,000 Hertz (Hz) and is greatest in the higher frequency. When the hearing loss exceeds 35 decibels (db) a hearing aid should be prescribed. This often improves communication but many old people are reluctant to use such an instrument. They may be diffident about admitting they are deaf, or have difficulty in learning the rather complex technique involved in using the instrument. Batteries may go flat. Hideous whines may occur when inadequate fitting allows sounds to be transmitted back from the earpiece to the receiver and there may be difficulty in adjusting the instrument to pick up conversation while keeping background noise to a minimum.

It is unfortunate that although there has been a major expansion in the provision of hearing aids, much less attention has been given to training patients in their use. Careful instruction on the use of the aid is essential, and regular follow-ups are important if effective use of the aid is to be achieved. In the absence of such formal education, doctors, nurses and relatives must take on the task of helping and encouraging old people to use their aids. Many old people can learn to lip read and should be taught

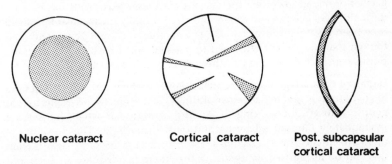

Nuclear cataract      Cortical cataract      Post. subcapsular cortical cataract

Figure 6.1   Types of cataract occurring in old age

this whenever possible, but unfortunately lip reading is another subject which has been neglected in planning therapeutic services for the elderly deaf and few formal teaching classes are held.

The recent appointment of a Hearing Therapist in the Southampton Health District has proved a great boon. Not only has she played an important part in the education and counselling of the elderly deaf, but she has trained and organised volunteers to do this. As a result many elderly have been helped at a relatively low cost.

## Vision (Case 1)

**Presbyopia.** Ageing is invariably accompanied by deteriorating vision, in which changes in the elasticity and translucency of the lens play an important part. Reduced elasticity interferes with accommodation so that, though distance vision remains intact, close vision becomes blurred. The change develops quite rapidly in early middle age, but can be corrected by fitting concave lenses.

**Cataract** (Case 5). Lens opacities tend to develop with age. A variety of patterns may be produced (Fig 6.1). The process is a consequence of ageing but it may be accelerated in some conditions (eg. diabetes, in which cataracts may develop in middle rather than old age).

Lens extraction is the only effective treatment. After the operation, considerable care must be taken to balance vision between the treated and untreated eyes with appropriate glasses. An alternative is to wait until vision is diminished in both eyes before operating. In the elderly, however, the waiting period may be sufficient to tip the balance between independence and permanent dependence. Operating on one eye, thereby providing the patient with monocular vision, is not a good solution. These problems should be resolved by the increasingly standard practice of performing bilateral extractions at an early stage. Pebble glasses provided to correct the visual defect after lens extraction may be difficult to get used to and cause confusion initially. Intraocular lens have now been greatly improved and are preferable. It should be remembered though that the patient will need to use eye drops regularly to keep his pupils constricted and the prosthetic lens from dislocating.

**Impaired dark adaptation.** Retinal changes make it difficult for old eyes to adapt from bright to dark surroundings, which creates problems for old people who go out walking or driving at night, or where houses are inadequately illuminated by natural or artificial light. The disability is often accentuated by a defective sense of balance. Domestic hazards from this can be minimised by ensuring that there is adequate artificial and natural lighting and that unseen hazards such as loose bannisters, worn steps, trailing flexes, torn vinyl floor covering, loose rugs, highly polished floors or children's toys, are avoided or corrected.

**Glaucoma.** Chronic simple glaucoma is a disease characterised by an increase in the pressure of fluid within the eyeball. Although ageing itself does not increase intraocular pressure, simple glaucoma has a peak incidence in the elderly. Table 6.1 summarises the features of the disease. Since the condition develops slowly, the patient often does not notice a gradual loss of peripheral vision. He may only notice that something is wrong when macular damage prevents him from focusing on objects by which time the visual change may be irreversible.

Table 6.1   Features of Chronic Simple Glaucoma

| | |
|---|---|
| Insidious onset | Central field defects |
| Reduced visual acuity | Macula not affected until late |
| Cupping of optic disc | Increased intraocular pressure |
| Optic nerve atrophy | |

Ideally, glaucoma should be identified as early as possible. Visual impairment should never be attributed to old age. All people involved in the care of the elderly should make sure that any deterioration in eyesight is reported and adequately investigated. Delay may be catastrophic.

The investigation and treatment of glaucoma is a task for the ophthalmic surgeon. Other doctors should help by not prescribing drugs likely to aggravate the condition. In general, any agent which dilates the pupil is likely to increase intraocular pressures and many of the drugs used in the elderly have this side effect; they include tranquillisers, bladder relaxants and anti-depressants. Clear communication between general practitioner, ophthalmologist, geriatrician, nurse, patient and relative is essential if disaster is to be avoided.

**Macular degeneration** (Case 2).   Old people may complain that while they are aware of their general surroundings they have great difficulty in seeing objects clearly. In other words, while they can find their way around the house, reading or watching television is impossible. These symptoms are often due to destruction of the macula, the part of the retina responsible for focusing onto fine detail. The condition is due to disease of local retinal blood vessels. If identified at a pre-symptomatic stage the condition can be arrested by photocoagulation of the offending blood vessels, but once vision has become impaired treatment is unlikely to be effective. People rarely present to an ophthalmologist at a pre-symptomatic stage, but close follow-up of patients with unilateral damage should ensure the early detection and treatment of the disease on the initially healthy side. Patients should be warned to report any deterioration in vision to their doctor immediately. Photocoagulation, if needed, should be done urgently within a short time of the deterioration. A delay of two weeks may mean that vision will be permanently affected. Some patients with more advanced disease benefit from wearing strong reading glasses or using a magnifying glass.

**Vascular disease.**   This is a common cause of visual loss. Any part of the eye's circulation may be affected, retinal, choroidal or the more posterior part. The loss may be transient – amaurosis fugax, or permanent. Occlusion of the arterial system causes a denser loss of vision than the venous system. While embolism is a common cause underlying conditions such as diabetes, hypertension, raised intracranial pressure, cranial arteritis (Chapter 7), glaucoma or migraine may exist. Treatment should be directed towards the underlying cause.

## Mobility

Many old people complain of decreased mobility with increasing age. Examination often reveals muscle wasting and weakness which is due in part to the progressive death of nerve cells controlling skeletal muscle movement. Unlike simpler cells, neurones cannot reproduce themselves and when cells die they are not replaced and function inevitably declines.

In parallel with this there is a reduction in the speed with which nerves conduct stimuli, and because nerves relaying position sense are involved old people often experience difficulty in maintaining their balance. Although ageing does interfere with muscle power and balance, a careful search should always be made for neurological disease (Table 6.2 *see also* Chapter 8).

Table 6.2   Neurological Causes of Immobility in the Elderly

| | |
|---|---|
| Cerebral lesions: | cerebrovascular accidents<br>Parkinsonism<br>advanced senile dementia<br>cerebral tumours |
| Mid-brain lesions: | vertebrobasilar insufficiency |
| Cord lesions: | cord ischaemia<br>$B_{12}$ and folate deficiency<br>meningioma<br>vertebral secondaries<br>tabes dorsalis |
| Peripheral nerve lesions: | neoplasms<br>diabetes<br>$B_{12}$ and folate deficiency<br>drugs |

Loss of articular cartilage is probably a natural consequence of ageing. When it is associated with thickening of the underlying bone and bone formation at the joint margins (osteophytes) osteoarthritis is considered to be present (Chapter 7), but it may not be the only locomotor cause of disability in old age (Table 6.3).

Table 6.3   Locomotor Causes of Immobility in the Elderly

| Structure | Disorder | |
| --- | --- | --- |
| Bone: | osteomalacia<br>Paget's disease<br>osteoporosis | myeloma<br>bony secondaries<br>fractures |
| Joint: | osteoarthritis<br>rheumatoid arthritis<br>'Charcot' joint | vascular necrosis of femoral<br>head<br>hallux valgus |
| Muscles: | 'fibrositis'<br>polymyalgia rheumatica<br>'lumbago' | |
| Foot: | corns<br>abnormal growth of toenails<br>(onychogryphosis) | ischaemic ulcers<br>deformities of the feet<br>(pes cavus, equinovarus, etc.) |

The previous paragraphs provide evidence that ageing is almost inevitably associated with some decline in neuromuscular performance. This is relatively minor and rarely if ever interferes with self-care capacity, so that someone experiencing difficulty in supporting herself at home is not suffering from old age, but from disease. This is sometimes curable, often treatable and always alleviable, and early identification of the problem is essential if loss of independence is to be avoided. This is only possible if all members of the health care team, including relatives, exercise a high degree of vigilance and suspicion.

## Mental function

**Mental impairment.**   There is considerable debate on whether or not ageing interferes with mental function. An apparent decline is often due to a communication problem, or a catastrophic change in the social situation (Table 6.4). The first essential in dealing with apparent mental frailty is to ensure that the patient is obtaining adequate input by correcting visual or hearing defects. Allowance must also be made for speech defects, for incoherence is often related to dysarthria or dysphasia rather than mental impairment. Confusion may also be compounded by a wide range of physical disorders. Chapter 9 gives more detailed consideration to this topic.

Table 6.4   Social and Communication Problems Producing Apparent Confusion

| Social problems | Communication problems |
| --- | --- |
| Change in housing | Deafness |
| Admission to residential care | Visual impairment |
| Admission to hospital | Dysphonia |
| Bereavement | Dysphasia |
| Family leaving home | Dysarthria |

**Depression.**   There is a striking rise in the incidence of depression in old age for reasons which have not yet been fully defined. Changes in the anatomy or biochemistry of the brain may be important but physical ill health, bereavement and a deteriorating social background often exert a major influence on the severity of depression.

The pain and deprivation caused by chronic illness is often sufficient in itself to cause depression. Traditional teaching is that anti-depressants are only of value where depression is the consequence of an intrinsic change in brain function. Practical experience suggests that this is not the case. Many lonely and disabled old people who are depressed respond extremely well to appropriate drug therapy.

A wide range of social stresses may contribute to depression. Bereavement (Chapter 15) has already been mentioned, but other less dramatic causes of isolation may contribute to depression including the marriage of children, the movement of children to a job in another part of the country, or rehousing away from a familiar neighbourhood.

Retirement may also be a time of stress, because within 24 hours a man may lose workmates, suffer a precipitous fall in income, lose his major source of interest and relinquish the family position of breadwinner. It may seem that his useful life has ended and that he has become a burden on society, and although this extreme reaction is relatively uncommon there is need for the more widespread development of pre-retirement courses (Chapter 4).

There are many less well-defined reasons for elderly people being depressed. Modern society tends to devalue the rôle of age in industry and recreation. Experience is considered to be less important than vitality and originality and this engenders a sense of inferiority which is accentuated by low incomes and inadequate housing.

**Poor nutrition** (Case 7)

Hospital staff are often shocked at the poor level of nutrition in many patients coming into their wards. This has given rise to a lot of public concern, and several large-scale community surveys have been organised which have found that most old people eat surprisingly well and that sub-nutrition, when it does occur, is usually associated with severe mental or physical incapacity. Social disadvantages are rarely the sole cause of sub-nutrition but they frequently exacerbate it in a co-existent medical disorder. Adverse factors include isolation, poverty and inadequate housing.

Old people are deficient of a wide range of nutrients but relatively few of these are important (Table 6.5), the exceptions being ascorbic acid and potassium. Ascorbic acid deficiency seriously interferes with wound healing, and is often responsible for a delayed recovery from an operation or the further breakdown of a pressure area. Potassium depletion due to a combination of poor diet and diuretic therapy may be responsible for profound muscle weakness. This might be avoided by ensuring that all old people on diuretics get *and take* potassium supplements.

The question of sub-nutrition and mental function remains unresolved.

Table 6.5    Nutrient Deficiency Related to Clinical Signs

| Nutrient | Clinical effect of deficiency | Importance of effect in old age |
|---|---|---|
| Thiamine | cardiac failure | minor |
| | peripheral neuritis | minor |
| Riboflavine | mouth and tongue changes | minor |
| Nicotinic acid | confusion | uncertain |
| | skin pigmentation | minor |
| | tongue changes | minor |
| | diarrhoea | minor |
| Pyridoxine | anaemia | minor |
| Folate | mental impairment | uncertain |
| | tongue changes | minor |
| | diarrhoea | minor |
| | cord and peripheral nerve degeneration | uncertain |
| Ascorbic acid | delayed wound healing (wounds include surgical scars, pressure areas, varicose ulcers) | major |
| Vitamin D | bone decalcification | uncertain |
| Iron | tiredness and lethargy | minor |
| Potassium | cardiac irritability | major |
| | muscle weakness | moderate |
| | depression | moderate |
| | mental impairment | moderate |
| Protein | loss of muscle mass | uncertain |
| | fluid retention | minor |
| Magnesium | alkaline urine | minor |
| Zinc | delayed wound healing | uncertain |

*Note:* this table refers to the situation as encountered in Great Britain; it may be different in countries where severe nutritional deficiency is common

The two conditions often co-exist in the same individual, but it is extremely difficult to separate cause from effect. Few studies have shown objective evidence that most confused old people benefit from vitamin supplements. Nonetheless, the theoretical possibility of improving the situation is such that many doctors prescribe either oral or parenteral supplements for confused, emaciated patients.

Recently, deficiency in trace elements such as zinc and copper has been suggested as being of importance in old age. While zinc deficiency may play a part in delaying wound healing there is little evidence for a clinical syndrome of zinc deficiency. Evidence also exists that vitamin and protein-calorie malnutrition are associated with a deficient immune response. While this may explain the lack of response to treatment of the undernourished, there is little evidence that the altered immune responses of ageing are due to sub-nutrition.

The first essential in improving the nutrition of old people is to identify who is at risk (Fig. 6.2). This is dependent upon good communication between doctors, nurses, social workers, neighbours, and relatives. People

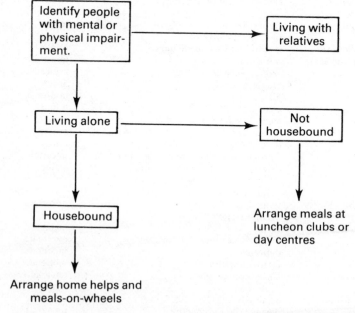

Figure 6.2  Allocation of resources for preventing subnutrition in the elderly

who are reasonably mobile are best managed at day centres or luncheon clubs, the inevitable social interaction playing an important part in stimulating an appetite.

Table 6.6   Consequences of Obesity

| | |
|---|---|
| Osteoarthritis | Hypertension |
| Gallbladder disease | Cardiac failure |
| Hiatus hernia | Accentuated respiratory failure |
| Reduced carbohydrate tolerance | Immobility and its consequences, |
| Coronary artery disease | ie. venous thrombosis, constipation |
| Cerebrovascular disease | and pressure sores |
| Peripheral vascular disease | |

Housebound patients have to rely on meals-on-wheels supplemented by the cooking and shopping efforts of relatives. A meals-on-wheels service will only be effective if it is directed to people in need; if it contains a good balance of nutrients; if nutrients are not destroyed by overheating; if meals are supplied every day or at least five times a week; and if the meals are sufficiently appetising for people actually to eat them. Good professional advice and careful co-ordination of voluntary and statutory organisations are necessary to achieve these objectives. Even when this exists it must be remembered that old people in receipt of meals-on-wheels will only get one meal. This is not totally sufficient for their needs and supplementation will be necessary.

Sub-nutrition effects a comparatively small section of the elderly population. Much more attention should be directed to over-nutrition. Obesity kills old men, immobilises old women and drives relatives to despair. Table 6.6 lists some of its more important complications. The only effective treatment is a reduction of food intake and because of the inactivity of the elderly this will need to be as low as 600 calories daily, a level which many old people will reject. Moral support and gentle bullying from both relatives and professionals is essential if weight loss is to be achieved, and particular attention must be paid to the control of edible gifts from well-meaning visitors at both home and hospital.

## Fatigue

It has long been accepted that decreased physical work capacity is an inevitable consequence of ageing. Important factors include the reductions in muscle power, in cardiac output and in pulmonary ventilatory capacity demonstrable in most old people. It is encouraging to note, however, that recent work from America and the Soviet Union suggests that many of these processes can be prevented or reversed by carefully graded exercise programmes. Confirmation of these observations could lead to a general introduction of physical education for the elderly and, ultimately, to a major decline in the high incidence of ill health and disability in this group.


## Skin changes

Changes in the skin and its integuments often provide the clearest evidence that an individual is ageing. The epidermis, dermis, hair follicles, melanocytes and exocrine and sebaceous glands are all affected by the passage of time.

A decline in the epithelial cell reproduction rate causes thinning of the epidermis and a reduction in sweat glands and sweat secretion. These factors combine to make the skin of old people dry and fragile and a variety of disorders may result.

There may be an intolerable itch (pruritus). Changes of temperature induced by undressing, going outdoors or taking a bath may be sufficient to trigger this off. Minor trauma related to woolly underwear may also initiate it and in more severe cases itching may be accompanied by small patches of scaling and redness. The symptom can be controlled by using bath oils and cold creams to keep the skin moist and avoiding extremes of temperature and rough clothing.

Local changes in the skin and a general reduction in immunological mechanisms increase the susceptibility of old people to skin infections. Fungal and, in particular, monilial infections can be particularly troublesome, the organism often attacking areas of skin already damaged by other factors. Nurses having difficulty in clearing up a breast intertrigo, or a urine rash should always consider this possibility and seek medical advice, for treatment with an appropriate anti-fungal cream will often solve the problem.

One of the few structures to hypertrophy with increasing age are sebaceous glands. Excess sebaceous secretion often produces an itchy, red and scaly rash which starts in the scalp and extends downwards to involve the neck, shoulders and chest. It can be controlled by regular washing with a cleansing agent such as cetrimide (Seboderm).

Ageing causes a reduction in the number of skin pigment cells, which accounts for the greying hair and skin pallor found in many old people. Along with an overall decline there may be local areas of pigment cell proliferation. This can produce a striking form of freckling involving exposed surfaces such as the forearm. It is of no clinical significance.

Old people exhibit a diffuse reduction in the density of hair follicles both on the scalp and on the rest of the body. Occasionally, the condition is a result of thyroid or vitamin C deficiency but it is quite distinct from the localised hereditary baldness which comes on at an early stage in many males.

## Further reading

Blazer D G (1982) *Depression in Late Life*. St Louis: Mosby

Comfort A (1979) *The Biology of Senescence*. Edinburgh: Churchill Livingstone

Ebrahim S B J, Sainsbury R & Watson S (1981) Foot problems of the elderly: a hospital survey. *Br Med J*, **283**, 949–950

Exton-Smith A N & Caird F I (1980) *Metabolic and Nutritional Disorders in the Elderly*. Bristol: Wright

Gardner D L (1983) The nature and causes of osteoarthritis. *Br Med J*, **286**, 418–424

Hinchcliffe R (1983) *Hearing and Balance in the Elderly*. London: Churchill Livingstone

Lamb M J (1977) *The Biology of Ageing*. Glasgow: Blackie

Marks R (1983) *Geriatric Dermatology*. London: Update Publications

Panel on Nutrition of the Elderly (1979) *A Nutrition Survey of the Elderly*. London: HMSO

Schaw R L, Christenses J M, Hutchinson, S M & Nerborne M A (1978) *Communication Disorders of the Aged*. Baltimore: University Park Press

# CHAPTER 7

# The Musculoskeletal System

### Muscles

It is a universal observation that increasing age is associated with a decline in muscle power (Fig. 7.1). A major factor in this is muscle atrophy due to the death of progressive numbers of the nerves in the spinal cord which activate muscles. This process starts very early in life, but at this stage surviving nerves sprout extra axon branches to re-innervate recently

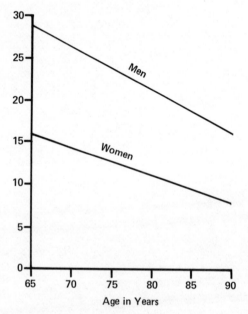

Figure 7.1   Grip strength in kg

denervated muscle fibres. Eventually, however, the task becomes too great for surviving nerves so that in old age there is a striking reduction in power.

This is only part of the story. Another reason for declining strength in old age is reduced physical activity. This has been demonstrated graphically in industrial workers who within a few months of retirement showed a dramatic decline in thigh muscle mass. Diet also is important. Sick old people may not eat sufficient protein to meet muscle requirements and this leads to further muscle wasting. The message then is that ageing does produce a decline in strength, but that this can be minimised by indulging in regular exercise, and taking a well-balanced diet.

## Myopathies

Despite the effects of ageing, healthy old people should be fully mobile and able to perform self-care activities. In the absence of joint or neurological disease, an old person who has difficulty in walking or getting out of a chair is likely to be suffering from a muscle disease (myopathy). Most of the conditions listed in Table 7.1 can be treated by dietary replacement or drug manipulation. These measures, however, are likely to be ineffective

Table 7.1   Causes of Myopathic Syndromes

| | |
|---|---|
| Hyperthyroidism | Steroid excess |
| Hypercalcaemia | Hypothyroidism |
| Hyperaldosteronism | Carcinomatosis |
| Hypokalaemia | Vitamin D deficiency |

unless the patient is put on to a rehabilitation programme. In vitamin D deficiency, for example, there is gross weakness of the thigh muscles, so that hip flexion exercises by the physiotherapist, reinforced by the nursing staff encouraging mobilisation, are essential if the patient is to make progress.

## Muscle pain

**General.**   Muscle pain due to unaccustomed exercise, exposure to cold, or psychological stress are common in all age groups, and usually respond to reassurance and treatment with a mild analgesic. The great danger in old age is that patients and sometimes their doctors attribute aches and pains to 'rheumatism' or 'fibrositis' without adequate investigation, thereby missing serious and often potentially treatable underlying disorders.

**Polymyalgia rheumatica.**    This is a disorder characterised by severe pain and stiffness of the shoulder and pelvic girdles. Examination usually reveals tenderness of the affected muscles, and the diagnosis is usually confirmed by finding a high erythrocyte sedimentation rate (ESR). The diagnosis is a rewarding one to make in that the patient responds dramatically to steroids and often within a matter of days is pain-free and fully mobile.

Another important reason for making the diagnosis is that the condition often is associated with inflammation of the cranial arteries (giant cell arteritis). The disorder usually can be identified by feeling tender and swollen temporal arteries, but sometimes this sign is missing. If the retinal or cerebral arteries are involved the patient may suffer sudden loss of vision in one eye or develop a stroke (Chapter 6). Steroid therapy, again, is effective in controlling the condition and preventing complications.

The starting dose of steroids should be high, say 30 mg of prednisolone daily. Once symptoms have settled, and once the erythrocyte sedimentation rate has fallen steroid dosage should be reduced gradually to maintenance levels of between 5 and 10 mg of prednisolone daily. Treatment should be continued for three years or even longer, being modified during this time in the light of changes in the erythrocyte sedimentation rate.

## Muscle cramps

Muscle cramps are common and often quite disabling. They tend to occur during the night and may be so disturbing as to cause severe depression, occasionally leading to suicide. The cause is not always obvious and in the majority of patients none can be found. Cramps may be associated with vitamin deficiency, uraemia, peripheral vascular disease or neurological disability. The drugs used for this condition are legion and more than one may need to be tried before success is achieved. Quinine sulphate, diazepam and orthoxine are probably the most successful, although often the only relief is to get up and to make a cup of tea; another remedy is to raise the head of the bed on blocks of wood or bricks. If these measures are unsuccessful, anti-convulsants, anti-depressants and vasodilators can be tried. (Epilepsy in the elderly may present as attacks of unilateral pain without convulsions – Chapter 8).

## Joint disease

**Ageing of joints.**    Articular cartilage, especially that involved in weight-bearing joints, undergoes changes throughout life from about the age of 25 years onwards. The material becomes more opaque, firmer and yellowish in colour and is less elastic and more resistant to deformation.

Defects, including clefts and ulcers, appear in the surface and increase in frequency and severity with advancing age. Above the age of 60 mucoid degeneration and cyst formation in the matrix is apparent, and calcification of articular cartilage, especially in the knee, occurs. The synovial membrane becomes denser and more thickened with villous hypertrophy, while in articular cartilage, there is an increase in the ratio of collagen to chondroitin sulphate with an overall reduction in the amount of chondroitin. Sclerosis and occlusion of capsular arterioles leading to local vascular insufficiency is associated with these changes.

## Osteoarthritis

Many of the changes found in ageing joints are found also in osteoarthritis. This is characterised by loss of articular cartilage, thickening of the underlying bony surfaces, and expansion of bone around the edges of the joint (osteophyte formation). Conditions listed in Table 7.2 accelerate these changes. Although joint changes are almost universal in old age

Table 7.2   Conditions Predisposing to Osteoarthritis

| | |
|---|---|
| Obesity | Rheumatoid arthritis |
| Trauma | Gout |
| Meniscectomy | Excessive use |
| Perthes disease | |

only a minority of subjects suffer symptoms. This has led to speculation that symptoms are related to inflammation rather than simple joint degeneration. The finding of high concentrations of irritant hydroxyapatite crystals in the joints of patients, and their favourable response to anti-inflammatory drugs, lends credence to this view.

## Hips and knees

In generalised osteoarthritis the interphalangeal joints of the fingers usually are involved. However, the hips and knees are the joints in which the disease causes most pain and disability. Flexion and extension of the knee is painful, and often is accompanied by a grating sensation (crepitus). The diagnosis of hip involvement may be more difficult in that pain often may be referred to the knee. Hip flexion, again, may be normal and pain only produced by external and internal rotation.

Treatment should aim at controlling pain and improving mobility. The first problem should be tackled by using one of the many non-steroidal anti-inflammatory drugs currently available. One of several which combine efficacy with safety is ibuprofen. Local treatment such as ice, heat or diathermy produces temporary alleviation of discomfort, but little long-term benefit. The physiotherapist is better occupied preventing muscle wasting and contractures by arranging active and passive exercises. Relatives and nursing staff should back this up by encouraging the patient to walk rather than be wheeled or carried during his day-to-day activities. Another obvious target is obesity, and here advice reinforced by gentle bullying by a dietician is useful. The place where diagnosis and treatment can be deployed most effectively is the day hospital, where staff can work out an overall strategy modifying this in the light of information on function at the hospital and in the patient's own home (Chapter 5).

## Joint replacement

Where osteoarthritis is particularly crippling, surgery should be considered. Total replacement of the hip with a ball-and-socket prosthesis can be very useful. For the operation to be a success, however, the patient should want the operation, be fit enough both to withstand it and to mobilise himself afterwards, and be alert enough to cooperate in a rehabilitation programme. Replacement of the knee joint is not such an established procedure in the elderly. It may be the only way of restoring mobility, however, particularly where there is gross joint deformity such as genu valgum. The simpler operation of patellectomy also may be helpful.

## Vertebral column

Degeneration of connective tissue in the inter-vertebral discs, and destruction of cartilage in the posterior (apophyseal) joints often conspire to produce severe back pain in old age. Prior to organising treatment for back pain, it is essential that diagnoses other than osteoarthritis are excluded. These are listed in Table 7.3. Again, evidence of root compression, such as sciatica, should be sought. A particularly insidious form of nerve compression is that involving the cauda equina, causing numbness

Table 7.3  Causes of Back Pain

| | |
|---|---|
| Muscle trauma | Multiple myeloma |
| Osteoarthritis | Tuberculosis |
| Prolapsed disc | Gastric disease |
| Vertebral trauma | Pancreatic disease |
| Osteoporosis/osteodystrophy | Renal disease |
| Secondaries | Herpes Zoster |

of the buttocks and incontinence of urine and faeces. If surgical treatment is to be effective the condition must be identified at an early stage.

Where the dorsal or lumbar vertebrae are involved, treatment with

Table 7.4   General Exercises for the Osteoarthritic Elderly Patient Whose Inter-
vertebral Joints are Involved

---

1   Slump down in chair. Go limp, then straighten spine to full (sitting) height slowly. Repeat 3 or 4 times.
2   Rock forward toward toes. Lift legs with bent knees from the ground for a count of 5 then lower slowly alternating legs. Slap feet on floor, first slowly then more quickly.
3   Press right then left arm alternately on chair arms, taking as much weight as possible.
4   Shrug shoulders up to ears several times. Rotate head slowly right and left several times.

---

non-steroidal anti-inflammatory analgesics should be coupled with advice on sleeping on a firmer mattress, and exercises designed to increase local mobility and relieve spasm (Table 7.4). Surgical corsets are best avoided in that they result in muscle wasting, are difficult to put on, and thus at the end of the day, increase rather than decrease dependence.

Osteoarthritis in the neck (cervical spondylosis) presents a more complex problem since, in addition to causing neck pain, it may be associated with spinal cord compression, nipping of nerve roots and compression of the vertebral arteries. A popular remedy is the cervical collar, but this tends to be loose fitting and useless, or well fitting and uncomfortable. There is little evidence that it produces long-term benefit in terms of pain relief, although by fixing the neck it may prevent attacks of dizziness due to kinking of the vertebral arteries. More drastic remedies such as traction rarely are applicable in the elderly.

Damage to the apophyseal joints interferes with the function of mechanoreceptors sited there. This results in the mid-brain and medulla being supplied with inadequate information on the position of the neck, so that the patient experiences symptoms of vertigo, unsteadiness and dizziness. Balance also may be impaired by direct compression of the spinal cord from osteophytes around the vertebral disc. Again, falls may be the result of brain stem ischaemia associated with compression of the vertebral arteries with osteophytes. There is increasing evidence, however, that these last two conditions are relatively rare causes of dizziness and unsteadiness, and that even the apparently classic picture of vertigo associated with sudden movements of the neck is more likely to be the result of apophyseal mechanoreceptor degeneration than either cord compression or vertebral artery stenosis.

## Shoulder movement

Diminished shoulder movement may be the result of osteoarthritis, but more usually when only a single joint is involved it is caused by inflammation of the joint capsule. This most commonly occurs after a stroke when, in the early stages, loss of support from muscles of the shoulder puts excessive strain on joint ligaments. It is best avoided by ensuring after a stroke that at all times the arm and forearm are supported. At the same time, passive and active exercises should be employed to keep the joint mobile. Once developed, the condition should be treated with local exercise, but often it proves extremely refractory to treatment. Local injections of hydrocortisone or the systemic administration of griseofulvin occasionally may help.

## Rheumatoid arthritis

When rheumatoid arthritis is encountered in old people it usually has been present since youth or middle age. It frequently is associated with severe deformity such as subluxation of the metacarpophalangeal joints, fixed shoulders, flexion deformities of the knees, gross deformity of the feet and dislocation of the atlanto-axial joint. This type of patient presents a particular challenge to the occupational therapist who has to maximise the few remaining capacities. In the intelligent patient, gadgetry ranging from lazy tongs to an electric wheelchair or to a POSSUM can make a major difference to his quality of life. It is to be hoped that in the future recent advances in drug therapy and surgery will reduce the number of such severely crippled patients presenting at the geriatric unit.

Less commonly, rheumatoid arthritis develops for the first time in old age. Characteristically, the onset is abrupt with intense joint pain and severe systemic effects such as pyrexia, nausea and rigors. The ESR is extremely high, and specific serological tests for rheumatoid factors are positive. Despite the dramatic onset the prognosis often is excellent and the patient may completely recover in one to two years.

Drug treatment of rheumatoid arthritis is essentially that for any age, but side effects increasingly dominate the picture. Examples include tinnitus and blood loss associated with salicylates, confusion and fluid retention with indomethacin, and osteoporosis and broken bones with corticosteroids. For similar reasons, penicillamine or immunosuppressant drugs should be used with caution in old age.

The therapeutic strategy varies with the prejudices of the clinician, but a reasonable approach might be to commence with standard doses of ibuprofen, and where this fails try one of the other non-steroidal anti-inflammatory agents. Where these fail to produce remission, second line therapy should be considered. After a long eclipse gold, as sodium aurithomaleate, has become increasingly popular. Side effects such as skin rashes, proteinuria, or marrow failure can be minimised by careful monitoring. Steroids may be used as a short course, starting with a high dose to produce a remission. Because of their adverse actions, steroids should be discontinued as soon as possible. If these all fail, the use of penicillamine should be considered.

## Gout and miscellaneous

Over 10 per cent of patients with gout experience their first attack after they have reached the age of 60 years. Standard methods of treatment and management of gout are used in elderly subjects, who tolerate well drugs such as probenecid and allopurinol. It is often the after-effects of gout that present problems by acting as a 'focus' for osteoarthritis.

Pseudogout (pyrophosphate arthropathy) is similar in many ways to classical gout but occurs more commonly in the elderly. The condition results from the formation of pyrophosphate crystals in the synovial fluid. It affects large joints, in particular the knee. Treatment and management are as for classical gout, although knee aspiration may abort the attack in the acute phase if swelling occurs. Patients with pseudogout should be investigated to exclude other diseases such as hyper-parathyroidism or haemochromatosis.

## Miscellaneous

Abnormal joints may be associated with neurological diseases such as tabes dorsalis, syringomyelia, or diabetic neuropathy, and may also result from the local treatment of a joint with intra-articular injections of a steroid or parenteral treatment with steroidal or non-steroidal anti-inflammatory agents. The joints are usually grossly deformed and enlarged, due to bony deformity as well as the effusion of fluid; instability may result and operation may be required to remedy this.

Infective arthritis is also common and although infection usually affects joints which already have been damaged by rheumatoid disease or osteoarthritis, normal joints may sometimes be involved. The usual infecting organisms are staphylococcus, streptococcus, gonococcus and meningococcus. Steroid therapy, given either systematically or by local intra-articular injections often predisposes to the development of the condition. Infective arthritis may give rise to systemic manifestations of septicaemia and, hence, in elderly patients presenting with systemic infections, joint infection should be excluded.

## Feet

Any assessment of the locomotor system should include a careful examination of the feet. Painful feet can severely interfere with mobility and lead to a progressive decline in physical capacity. Table 7.5 lists some of

Table 7.5   Common Foot Problems in the Elderly

| | |
|---|---|
| Corns | Peripheral ischaemia |
| Hammer toes | Trophic ulcer |
| Hallux valgus | Onychogryphosis |
| Bunions | (thickened nail) |
| Plantar wart | Fungal infection |

the more common conditions to be identified. Many of these problems require the skills of a chiropodist or even an orthopaedic surgeon, but simple measures such as advice on footwear, or help in clipping nails may be all that is required.

## BONES

### Bone ageing and osteoporosis

Bone mass increases rapidly up to adolescence and continues to increase at a reduced rate until the early 30s. In women, at the menopause there is a particularly rapid loss of bone for several years followed by a slower decline throughout the rest of life. In men, bone mass declines steadily from about the age of 45 onwards. There is wide individual variation. A massive reduction in bone mass after the menopause only occurs in some women, and many old men show little reduction in bone mass over 10 or 20 years. This means that only a minority of people develop bone rarefaction sufficiently severe to create practical problems.

Extreme rarefaction is described as osteoporosis. While this may occur as a result of ageing alone, a wide range of conditions can accentuate it (Table 7.6). Amongst the clinical manifestations of the disease is collapse of dorsal and lumbar vertebrae resulting both in a loss of height and a forward curvature of the spine (kyphosis). If the collapse is sudden it is associated with severe pain which eventually settles as the fracture

Table 7.6   Causes of Bone Rarefaction

| | |
|---|---|
| Ageing | Renal disease |
| Steroid therapy | Diabetes |
| Rheumatoid arthritis | Partial gastrectomy |
| Thyrotoxicosis | Reduced mobility |

heals. Other sites at risk are the lower end of the radius, particularly after the menopause in women, and through the neck of femur particularly in men and women over the age of 70. Investigations supporting clinical evidence of osteoporosis are radiological evidence of bone rarefaction, coupled with normal serum levels of calcium, phosphate and alkaline phosphatase.

Medical treatment of the condition remains unsatisfactory. The simplest and safest one is to give calcium gluconate (effervescent) in a dose of 1 gm three times daily. This, though not correcting rarefaction, prevents further calcium loss. Oestrogens are effective in post-menopausal women, but should not be used in the elderly. The anabolic steroid, stanozolol, may actually increase bone density, but preliminary findings need to be substantiated. Other régimes are either ineffective, or too complex or toxic for routine use.

The general management of osteoporosis poses problems. Severe back pain associated with vertebral collapse may be relieved by bed rest. If this is prolonged, however, the patient becomes immobile, and further bone loss is encouraged. The most satisfactory compromise is to treat the patient with severe pain with analgesics and a few days bed rest, but to follow this with progressively intensive mobilisation exercises. Spinal braces should be avoided since, by limiting vertebral movement, they encourage further skeletal rarefaction.

## Osteomalacia

In osteomalacia the mass of the skeleton remains the same, but there is progressive decalcification so that bones become soft, painful and liable to fracture. The condition is due to an inadequate absorption of calcium, resulting from deficiency of vitamin D, a substance essential for both the absorption of calcium, and the deposition of this in the skeleton.

The condition is particularly common in old people who are housebound. Part of the problem is that they have an inadequate intake of vitamin D. Even more important is that they are not exposed to sunlight. Sunlight increases vitamin D levels by converting precursors sited in the skin into the vitamin.

A patient with osteomalacia may present with bone pain or even a fracture. She also often has a waddling gait due to the fact that vitamin D deficiency causes weakness of the thigh muscles. X-rays show poorly calcified bones, and the serum calcium and phosphate concentrations are low, whereas that of the alkaline phosphatase is elevated. The diagnosis can, if necessary, be confirmed by demonstrating decalcified bone in a biopsy specimen.

Treatment consists of giving a single injection of 600,000 units of calciferol or an oral dose up to a maximum of 5,000 iu daily for 3 months. During this time a close watch should be kept on serum calcium levels since excessive calcium absorption can lead to kidney damage, vomiting and diarrhoea, and even mental impairment.

Many clinicians believe that florid osteomalacia merely is the tip of the iceberg, and that many more frail old people, although having normal serum calcium levels, suffer from vitamin D deficiency associated with skeletal decalcification. There may be a place then for supplementing the diets of housebound old people with vitamin D as say, calcium and vitamin D tablets 500 iu daily. Larger doses should be avoided because of the risks of hypercalcaemia.

## Paget's disease

Paget's disease of bone is characterised by an increase in the rate of bone turnover accompanied by remodelling of the bone contour. The cause is as yet unknown. Its incidence rises with increasing age, and it is estimated to be present in about 10 per cent of people over the age of 85 in the majority of whom the disease gives rise to no symptoms and is often only recognised following radiology for some other purpose.

The condition is important since it may give rise to the complications listed in Table 7.7. The most important of these are heart failure, bone pain, fractures, malignant change and deafness.

The most effective agent in the treatment of Paget's disease is calcitonin, a hormone extracted from the thyroid glands of animals. In Paget's disease its main effect is to diminish bone resorption and thus decrease bone turnover. Its principle use is in the relief of bone pain, but it may also be effective in promoting the rate of healing of fractures, in relieving deafness and in controlling high output cardiac failure. A satisfactory regime would be the injection of 100 MRC units of salmon calcitonin three days a week for three months, monitoring response by the disappearance of symptoms and a fall in an elevated serum alkaline phosphatase concentration.

Table 7.7   Complications of Paget's Disease of Bone

| |
| --- |
| Bone pain |
| Joint deformity → osteoarthritis |
| High output cardiac failure |
| Osteogenic sarcoma |
| Platybasia → deafness |
| Paraplegia |
| Deafness |
| Fractures |

### Fractured proximal femur

In old age there is a precipitous rise in the incidence of fractures of the proximal end of the femur (Fig. 7.2). This partly results from the high prevalence of disorders such as osteoporosis, osteomalacia and Paget's disease. Equally important is the increased risk of old people falling. Patients with fractures are more likely to be demented, to have poor vision, to have cerebrovascular disease or to suffer from drop attacks. General principles in the management of the condition include the following:

1 Surgical intervention is essential. Treatment with traction is useless, as it invariably produces permanent immobility in old people.
2 Patients should be thoroughly investigated for intercurrent medical disorders. An old lady will not get better if her cardiac failure, anaemia and diabetes remain untreated.

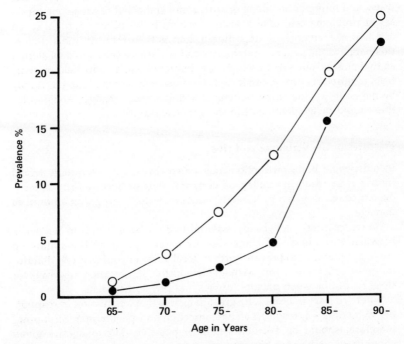

Figure 7.2   Prevalence of fractured proximal neck of femur in men ● and women ○
(Grimley-Evans 1979)

3 Secondary causes of the fracture should be excluded. Osteomalacia, cancerous deposits and Paget's disease will modify the surgical approach to the fracture.
4 A multi-disciplinary rehabilitation programme should be organised (Chapter 5).

It is obvious that the geriatric physician must be involved in the management of the patient from the outset. He will have little to offer if he is merely asked to dispose of patients who become stuck in orthopaedic beds. There is no doubt that when a combined geriatric/orthopaedic approach is adopted that bed turnover increases and patients benefit.

## Fractured wrist

Fractures of the distal radius and ulna reach their peak incidence in women immediately after the menopause, but remain common in old age. While in youth a broken wrist is painful and unpleasant, the situation in old age often is aggravated by the patient already being disabled in other ways, and living either alone or with a frail and elderly spouse or sibling. Major problems can arise if such a patient has a plaster applied in an accident and emergency department, and is then sent off home. Before this happens the general practitioner and social services should be alerted so that appropriate services such as a district nurse, a home help or visits from neighbours can be organised. In extreme situations, indeed, it may be necessary to admit the patient to hospital and, ideally, provision for this should be available within the geriatric service.

## Fractures of the vertebrae and ribs

In old people bone rarefaction may be so severe that seemingly trivial injuries may result in a collapsed vertebral body or fractured rib. Indeed, even a cough, a yawn or a hearty laugh may do a surprising amount of damage.

When treating a collapsed vertebral body a balance has to be struck between providing sufficient rest to relieve pain, and maintaining sufficient mobility to prevent further decalcification and to arrest deterioration in general function. Management of this injury, therefore, calls for close liaison between doctors, nurses and physiotherapists.

Where ribs are fractured the great danger is that a reduction in respiratory excursion will result in a chest infection and pneumonia. Strapping, therefore, should be avoided wherever possible. The analgesics given should strike a balance between relieving pain so that the patient is not afraid to take deep breaths, and over sedating so that respiration is impaired and an infection develops. The physiotherapist also has an important role in encouraging the maximum use of the thorax despite the considerable amount of discomfort involved in doing so.

Collapsed vertebrae or broken ribs fairly often are due to the blood-borne spread of tumour cells, and in this situation treatment with radiotherapy, cytotoxic drugs or hormones may have to be considered (Chapter 15).

### Further reading

Devas M (1977) *Geriatric Orthopaedics*. London: Academic Press

Dixon A S (1983) Non-hormonal treatment of osteoporosis. *Br Med J*, **286**, 999–1000

Gilchrist A K (1979) Common foot problems in the elderly. *Geriatrics*, **34**, November, 67–70

Hosking D J (1981) Paget's disease of bone. *Br Med J*, **283**, 686–688

Paterson C R & MacLennan W J (1984) *Bone Disease in the Elderly*. Chichester: Wiley

Stevenson J C & Whitehead M I (1982) Postmenopausal osteoporosis. *Br Med J*, **285**, 585–588

Wright V (1983) *Bone and Joint Disease in the Elderly*. Chichester: Wiley

# CHAPTER 8

# The Neurology of Old Age

The physician in geriatric medicine spends much of his time dealing with the ravages of neurological disease, often being called in to see the patient when 'nothing more can be done'. In some instances, such as Parkinson's disease, modern drug treatment has made it possible to use simple measures to revolutionise the life of the patient. In others, such as cerebrovascular disease, the path to improvement is harder and longer. Nonetheless, attention to detail in diagnosis and assessment, and the use of positive and modern rehabilitation techniques usually pay long term dividends in terms of mobility, self sufficency and self respect.

## Stroke illness

A stroke is a sudden ischaemic or haemorrhagic disorder of the brain, often resulting in a focal neurological deficit. It covers a wide spectrum ranging from transient focal signs such as weakness or loss of vision (transient ischaemic neurological attack), through gross unilateral weakness and sensory disturbance, to deep coma with severe disturbance to vital centres.

## Aetiology

Stroke due to blockage of the cerebral arteries or haemorrhage from a cerebral artery frequently is a manifestation of a more generalised arterial disease. There is increasing evidence that attention to a wide range of risk factors in atherosclerosis would reduce the likelihood of these catastrophes (Chapter 10).

Stroke illness may be conveniently divided into transient ischaemic neurological attacks (TIAs), recovered ischaemic neurological deficits (RIND) and completed strokes with a permanent neurological deficit.

## Transient ischaemic neurological attack

Warning of an impending stroke often may be given by a transient ischaemic attack. This usually results from debris, normally platelet clots, breaking away from an atheromatous ulcer or a damaged heart valve. These may block a retinal artery causing temporary blindness (amaurosis fugax) or may enter a cerebral artery causing transient weakness or sensory disturbance (TIA). In both these situations signs resolve within 24 hours.

The symptoms experienced by the patient will depend on the part of the brain affected and this in turn will depend on which arterial system supplies that part of the brain. Flow patterns from the carotid arteries will tend to produce hemiparetic symptoms, while those from the vertebral arteries will tend to affect the brain stem and posterior lobe of the cerebrum giving rise to dizziness, loss of balance or visual disturbance. It would seem that TIA's affecting the carotid system carry a worse prognosis for completed stroke than those affecting the vertebral/basilar system.

## Recovered Ischaemic Neurological Deficit (RIND)

In these cases, often called 'little strokes', the neurological deficit persists for more than 24 hours. Recovery of function is eventually complete though sometimes this will take days or even several weeks so that eventually no neurological deficit can be detected. As with TIAs, a RIND may be followed after an interval, or even several RINDs, by a completed stroke.

## Completed stroke

**Diagnosis.**    When a patient presents with weakness down the one side of his body, the first thing to do is to assess whether or not this represents a stroke. The weakness may be due to a primary or secondary tumour. Here the history of a slow, persistent but fluctuating deterioration is a useful clue. The distinction is important in that if the tumour is benign, surgery may be indicated. Even if the condition is malignant, treatment with high doses of the corticosteroid dexamethasone may reduce swelling and intracranial pressure, producing a temporary alleviation of symptoms. At worst, the diagnosis of malignancy saves the patient from the effort and frustration of intensive, but inappropriate, efforts to rehabilitate him.

Another diagnosis to be excluded is a subdural haemorrhage, in which damage to vessels in the dura mater results in a blood clot which compresses adjacent brain tissue. Clasically there is a recent history of head injury or a fall associated with an impaired, but fluctuating, level of consciousness. Sometimes, these clues may be absent so that a high index of suspicion is necessary if the diagnosis is not to be missed. Surgical drainage of the blood clot often produces complete remission of signs. A less common cause is inflammation of the arteries in conditions such as temporal arteritis (Chapter 7), disseminated lupus erythomatosis or polyarteritis nodosa.

**Assessment.** Once the diagnosis, cerebrovascular disease, is established, an assessment of the patient's previous functional capacity is a vital preliminary to treatment and rehabilitation. Otherwise, scarce resources may be misused and an exhausting and uncomfortable régime imposed on a patient who cannot improve. Moreover, an accurate initial assessment makes it easier to measure progress in response to treatment.

The first thing requiring evaluation is the patient's general condition. It may be that there is a long history of dementia, that there have been several previous strokes producing severe incapacity or that his exercise tolerance was restricted by severe cardiorespiratory disease.

A detailed evaluation should then be made of his present condition. Aspects of this are listed in Table 8.1. The most important of these is cognitive ability. Mental impairment will seriously impede any progress. Again, the patient must be motivated. If he is depressed, or sees little to be gained by increased mobility, he is unlikely to cooperate in a programme of rehabilitation.

Table 8.1　Changes in Function After a Stroke

| | |
|---|---|
| Mental impairment | Apraxia |
| Depression | Loss of position sense |
| Emotional lability | Astereognosis |
| Dysphasia | Agnosia |
| Dysarthria | Homonymous hemianopia |
| Dysphagia | Neglect of affected side |
| Muscle weakness | Denial of illness |
| Changed muscle tone | Changed bladder tonus |

Muscle power should be assessed (Table 8.2), but more important than this is evaluation of muscle tonus. A patient will be unable to stand on a flaccid leg, or have difficulty in using a spastic foot fixed in plantar flexion. Speech defects cause a great deal of frustration and can give rise to the patient being labelled wrongly as cantankerous, confused, or even unconscious. Visual impairment should be identified. Damage of pathways to the occipital cortex results in loss of vision to one side (homonymous hemianopia) and may account for a patient walking into things, or being unable to read properly.

Sensory abnormalities are easily missed, but seriously interfere with rehabilitation. If he has disturbed position sense, a patient will not know where his leg is and thus be unable to use it in walking (astereognosis).

Table 8.2   Grades Used in Assessing Recovery of Muscle Power

| | |
|---|---|
| Complete paralysis | 0 |
| Flicker of movement | 1 |
| Movement when gravity removed | 2 |
| Movement against gravity | 3 |
| Movement weak against resistance | 4 |
| Normal compared to unaffected side | 5 |

He may be unable to recognise the function of objects, and, to give an extreme example, attempt to write with a banana (agnosia); or unable to fit movements together in the correct sequence, and thus instead of walking remain rooted to the spot (apraxia). His image of himself and his body may be distorted so that he may not recognise that his limbs are paralysed, may not recognise them as part of himself, or may show complete neglect for one side of his body (denial). An extreme example of this is neglect of the world on the affected side. A doctor talking from the affected side will be ignored, but may be able to establish contact by going round to the other side. It is as though the doctor has gone through a door in the patient's consciousness. The patient will have difficulty in describing these abnormalities, so that he all too commonly gets labelled wrongly as being stupid, lazy, stubborn or even demented.

Once treatment is started, its efficacy should be evaluated regularly. The simplest way of doing this is to use a simple measure of disability (Table 8.3). If over several weeks there is little change in this, consideration has to be given as to whether the programme of rehabilitation needs to be changed or indeed whether targets need to be reset. An example may be that it will become clear that a patient will not be able to go home again, so that attention should be directed to getting him fit for residential

Table 8.3   Grades of Disability in Cerebrovascular Disease (Rankine 1957)

| | |
|---|---|
| Grade I: | No significant disability (able to carry out all usual duties) |
| Grade II: | Slight disability (unable to carry out previous activities, but able to look after affairs without assistance) |
| Grade III: | Moderate disability (requiring some help, but able to walk without assistance) |
| Grade IV: | Moderately severe disability (unable to walk without assistance and unable to attend own bodily needs without assistance) |
| Grade V: | Severe disability (bedridden, incontinent and requiring constant nursing care and attention) |

care. Again, it may be that long term hospital care will be necessary, so that the programme should be directed to preventing the adverse effects of institutionalisation (Chapter 9).

**Medical treatment.** The immediate management of a stroke is dependent on its severity. In the case of a TIA, treatment should be aimed at preventing the formation of platelet clots and emboli by reducing platelet stickiness. The simplest drug to use is aspirin given in a small dose, 75 or 150 mg may be sufficient, and this may be combined with dipyridamole in a dose of 100–200 mg three times a day. If the patient is relatively fit, has little other evidence of atherosclerosis, and has an identifiable source of the embolism, surgery either to a heart valve or a narrowed carotid artery should be considered.

Other underlying conditions associated with arteriosclerosis, such as diabetes mellitus (Chapter 11), hypertension (Chapter 10) and myxoedema (Chapter 11) should be sought and treated. This may be important in preventing further episodes producing either RIND or completed stroke. The value of preventing platelet aggregation in these two latter conditions remains yet to be proved, and the results of further trials of newer antiplatelet aggregating drugs in all these conditions need careful evaluation.

Antidepressants may be of value in the treatment of completed stroke. This is a very negative illness and the patient may well be affected by loss of function. Imipramine may also help to alleviate emotional lability. It must be remembered that it, and indeed all tricyclic antidepressants, have side effects, particularly postural hypotension, which may limit their use.

## Management of the acute phase

When a stroke is severe, measures initially should be directed at ensuring that the airway of the patient is not obstucted, that he is hydrated adequately, that he does not develop pressure areas, or a respiratory infection. In coma it may be necessary to insert an airway or endotracheal tube, and give intravenous fluids. If the patient is rousable his swallowing reflex should be checked, and where this is absent, a nasogastric tube passed ensuring that it really is in the stomach rather than the trachea. Assessment of fluid balance is difficult because a loss of thirst sensation and a lax inelastic skin often obscure dehydration. In this situation an input/output chart, measuring output by a urinary catheter may be necessary.

## The rehabilitation team

Once and indeed even before the clinical condition of the patient has stabilised, attention should be given to rehabilitation. This aspect of stroke management exemplifies particularly well the points made in Chapter 5 about the importance of close and planned communication and collaboration between all members of the therapeutic team in the care of elderly patients.

## The remedial therapists

Physiotherapy, initially at least, should aim at restoring function to the affected side rather than encouraging greater use of the unaffected side to the detriment of the other. Techniques for doing this vary. That used by Bobath involves reducing spasticity by developing movement patterns to counteract those involved in spasticity. A reduction in tonus is increased by tactile and proprioceptive stimuli. Again, mass movements are suppressed by encouraging selective muscle activity. When balancing, the patient is encouraged to use his paralysed side rather than merely depend upon the unaffected one. The rate at which patients progress varies a great deal so that if morale is to be maintained, it is important that each target set should be within the capacity of the patient, and that a fresh target should be set only when the initial one has been achieved. Exercises also should be of such a nature that their relevance to mobilisation and self sufficiency are obvious to the patient. An example is that he should not be asked to walk before he is able to sit up, and has been convinced that he is able to do this.

The occupational therapist works in parallel with the physiotherapist training the patient to wash, dress, feed and toilet himself. This may involve modifications to his clothing such as using adhesive Velcro in the place of buttons or zips, or replacing shoe laces with elastic. Modification to feeding and kitchen utensils also may be important. Close collaboration between occupational therapist and physiotherapist is necessary so that their training patterns reinforce rather than counteract each other.

A further important member of the rehabilitation team is the speech therapist. She is involved in the re-establishment of communication by dysphasic patients, in modifying movements of articulation for dysarthria and in retraining patients with reading difficulties (dyslexia). If attempts at retraining and writing problems (dysgraphia) are unsuccessful she is able at least to provide both patient and family with a realistic evaluation of his limitations, teaching them where appropriate to cope by means of such strategies as pictures or an Indian sign language.

## The nurse

In hospital, the person who spends most time with the patient is the nurse, and it is important that she should reinforce the training given by her colleagues. Examples are that patients should walk rather then be pushed to the lunch table; that they should dress themselves; and that the nurse should spend time talking to patients with speech difficulties. She also should be responsible for organising the patient's day so that self care activities, rehabilitation and recreation fit together in such a way that the interest of the patient is maintained, his motivation stimulated and undue fatigue avoided. Another important task is to observe and report back on progress to other members of the team.

If rehabilitation is well organised it can be expected that, of patients surviving the first three weeks of their illness, one quarter will be completely independent, half will be able to walk with an aid and require a limited amount of help with self care, while another quarter will remain chairfast and heavily dependent. Before the patient is discharged steps should be taken to ensure that his capacities are sufficient to cope with the environment to which he is returning. In some instances this will involve members of the rehabilitation team visiting his home so that structural adaptations can be arranged, and additional aids such as commodes, raised toilet seats or bath seats supplied.

## Discharge and follow-up

It is important to recognise that once patients with a stroke or any other major disability are discharged from hospital their condition may deteriorate. Over the course of a year, a large proportion will lose their mobility or become increasingly dependent. The general practitioner has an important part to play in ensuring effective medical follow-up with, where necessary, referral for further rehabilitation at a day hospital to maintain function and avoid future regression. The heavy physical and psychological pressures a stroke patient imposes on his family must be recognised. Even if a patient is mobile, the fact that his life style is limited to walking round the house and watching television, may make him frustrated, abusive and difficult to live with. It is important, therefore, not merely to treat the patient, but also to 'care for the carers'. One way of relieving the pressure is to organise a system whereby a team of volunteers provide a course of continued rehabilitation, diversion and entertainment. Speech therapists have led the way in devising such programmes.

The treatment of stroke illness in the elderly is one of the most demanding and challenging aspects of geriatric medicine. It requires the skilled interaction of a multi-disciplinary team, linking both the hospital and the community. The attitudes to the disease by the patient, his relatives and his therapists plays a vital part in his recovery. For the greatest success to be achieved all therapists must show realistic optimism. Recovery from a completed stroke is not instantaneous. Full rehabilitation is usually only achieved over a period of two or three months or even longer. For this reason the admission of stroke patients to an acute medical ward with a rapid tempo is often inappropriate. Several hospitals have special units specifically designed for the management of strokes; with the concentration of the necessary skills their results have been most encouraging.

## Parkinson's disease

The clinical manifestations of Parkinsonism are a combination of tremor, muscle rigidity and generalised poverty of movement (hypokinesia). The tremor is at its worst when the patient is relaxed and improves when he engages in purposeful activity. The rigidity is particularly disabling, the resistance produced by it being compared with that experienced when bending a lead pipe, but because of the associated tremor it is often jerky and called 'cog-wheel'. Poverty of movement manifests itself as an expressionless face, motionless arms and a shuffling gait. When the patient walks he is bent forward, holds his arms rigidly at his sides and rushes along with small shuffling steps (festination) in a perpetual battle to keep up with himself. Other symptoms include excessive salivation and an increased sebaceous gland secretion. At autopsy, loss of neurones can be identified in the basal nuclei and substantia nigra. This is accompanied by a gross reduction in dopamine, an important neurotransmitter.

Most cases are of unknown aetiology, but a substantial minority result from the use of phenothiazine tranquillisers which when used in the very old may unmask a subclinical deficiency of dopamine due to age. Alzheimer's disease and multi-infarct dementia also may present with akinesia and rigidity (Chapter 9). This condition usually can be distinguished from Parkinson's disease by virtue of the fact that tremor is absent, and that sufferers rarely respond to anti-Parkinsonian drugs.

The natural history of the disease is gradual progression over several years to a state of increased dependency and disability. Death usually results from a respiratory infection when a state of severe inanition is reached. Secondary, and by no means universal, features are those of mental impairment and endogenous depression. Damage to the autonomic nervous system also is common so that the patient dribbles excessive quantities of saliva and is at risk from postural hypotension (Chapter 10) and hypothermia (Chapter 13).

Treatment has been revolutionised by the use of levo-dopa. Following absorption, this reaches the central nervous system where it is converted into the neurotransmitter dopamine by the enzyme decarboxylase. The drug increases mobility, and reduces rigidity and tremor and often relieves co-incidental depression. Effective blood concentrations with fewer gastro-intestinal side effects can be achieved by combining the drug with an agent which prevents the metabolism of levo-dopa by enzymes in the gastro-intestinal mucosa. Levo-dopa does not arrest Parkinson's disease; it merely reduces the initial severity of the condition giving the patient a few more years of active life before he declines into a state of severe disability. Fortunately, perhaps, the drug often allows old people to live long enough to die from other diseases before Parkinsonism catches up with them.

It is important to start with small doses and gradually increase them, small changes in the elderly being made at least ten days apart. If adverse effects occur, the dose should be reduced and further tentative attempts made to increase it again after one month's stabilisation.

In about a fifth of patients L-dopa may produce an acute hallucinatory state, and when this happens there is no alternative but to cease therapy. Other patients may develop bizarre movements of their lips and tongue which are evidence of too high a blood level and easily controlled by reducing dosage.

If a state is reached where the condition of the patient deteriorates despite increased dosage of levo-dopa it is worth trying the dopamine receptor agonist bromocriptine. This drug is expensive and has many side effects and should thus be reserved for patients whose disease becomes resistant to levodopa. Bromocriptine is ineffective in patients who show an initial resistance to levodopa and should not be used in patients who are dementing.

The anticholinergic drugs remain an effective treatment in the early stage of the disease. Some (benztropine) tend to accumulate and all may give rise to confusional states. The antihistaminic orphenadrine (Disipal) and benzhexol (Artane) are the most used, but their wider anticholinergic side effects may make them inappropriate for use in some elderly. Finally, amantadine (Symmetrel) may also be useful in some patients. Its mode of action is uncertain. If it is going to relieve symptoms it will do so within a short time of starting treatment and it is not worth persevering with treatment if this is ineffective for more than four weeks, particularly as it will cause confusional states.

A newer introduction is selegiline (Eldepryl). This is a monoamine-oxidase-B inhibitor given in a dose of 5 mg which may be increased to 10 mg after an interval. When initiating treatment with this substance, it is wise to halve the current dose of levodopa and to wait several days to observe its effect before increasing levodopa dosage again. It may be useful in end-stage Parkinson's disease.

As the condition progresses drug treatment usually has to be supplemented by a course of rehabilitation. This is best conducted at the day hospital, where collaboration between doctor and physiotherapist can achieve the greatest degree of mobility for the simplest drug régimes. Inpatient treatment is associated with a high morbidity and mortality from respiratory infection: consequently, relatives should be warned of the risks of intermittent 'relief' hospital admissions should these prove necessary.

## Involuntary movements

Old people occasionally exhibit involuntary rapid jerking movements of their arms and legs. In a less extreme form the condition presents as purposeless mastication and lip smacking movements. The condition is embarrassing both to the patient and his relatives, but it is not associated with mental impairment and rarely causes severe incapacity. Though the nature of the disorder is far from clear it responds with varying success to drugs which block dopamine receptor sites in the brain. An example is chlorpromazine.

Slow writhing movements of the tongue, mouth and lips (tardive dyskinesia) are usually the result of a drug side effect. In psychotic patients it is associated with the use of massive doses of phenothiazine drugs. The underlying mechanism is thought to be blockage of dopamine receptors. Paradoxically, in old people the condition is more usually associated with levo-dopa therapy. In this situation appropriate reduction in dosage usually resolves the problem. Less commonly, other agents including oestrogens and the antiemetic metoclorpramide may be responsible.

## Tremor

Not all old people with tremor are suffering from Parkinson's disease. A substantial proportion have a senile tremor. In this the tremor may be either fine and rapid, or coarse and slow. It is absent at rest, and increased by emotion and voluntary movements. Though a source of inconvenience the condition is relatively innocuous in that it is not associated with akinesia or rigidity, and does not progress to severe incapacity. Characteristically, the condition is relieved by alcohol. A less addictive remedy is the beta blocking agent, propranolol.

## Falls

An old person who has recurrent falls is at risk from a wide range of conditions ranging from a fractured neck of femur to hypothermia. He is a source of concern to his relatives, who often seek institutionalisation, because they are afraid to leave him alone 'in case something happens'.

For these reasons it is essential that the causes for falls be identified and, where possible, the situation be remedied.

**Environment.**   The problem may be the patient's environment. Many old people live in houses with badly worn steps, wrongly sited bannisters, rooms with poor natural and artificial lighting, and cupboards, switches and coin operated meters accessible only by climbing on a chair. Others seem to delight in having long trailing flexes, wobbly furniture, highly polished floors, and loose carpets and mats. The general practitioner, district nurse or health visitor should be on the lookout for these hazards, and where appropriate, suggest diplomatically that the situation be altered. In some instances, this may involve private or local authority contractors in a considerable amount of reconstruction, and in extreme cases a move to more suitable housing may have to be suggested.

**Ageing.**   Ageing itself increases the risk of old people falling and Table 8.4 lists some of the reasons for this. The risk is even greater where ageing

Table 8.4   Effect of Ageing on Balance

| |
| --- |
| Visual impairment |
| Vestibular degeneration |
| Cervical apophysical joint degeneration |
| Impaired position sense |

is compounded with neurological disease. This may present in a variety of ways. It may be that the patient feels unsteady when on his feet. Amongst the more common causes for this is osteoarthritic degeneration of the cervical spine (Chapter 7).

## Vertigo

Another site which may be damaged is the inner ear vestibule. Causes for this include ischaemia, and Meniere's disease (a condition in which excessive quantities of fluid accumulate in the vestibule). In ischaemia the condition may respond to vasodilator such as betahistine hydrocholoride. Treatment with diuretics or even surgery may be necessary in Meniere's disease. Drugs which control dizziness by sedating the central nervous system work well in younger patients, but should be used with extreme caution in old age. They may reduce the sensation of unsteadiness, but by suppressing righting reflexes may increase the risk of falls. Prochlorperazine (Stemetil) is a frequently prescribed drug which may do more harm than good in this situation.

## Drop attacks

The patient may complain that when she falls her legs seem to just give way under her. She may then be suffering from 'drop attacks' a disorder more common in elderly women in which there are episodes where there is a sudden loss of postural tonus in the legs. The knees of the patient bend under her, and she finds herself on the ground unable to move her legs. Power only returns to her legs if she can press her feet against a solid surface. Sometimes the condition is due to a poor blood supply to the mid-brain, and is precipitated by sudden movements of the neck. More usually there is no clear-cut pathology.

## Epilepsy

In other patients, falls may be associated with a loss of consciousness. This may have a variety of causes. Epilepsy is high on the list, and here an eyewitness account from a relative may be useful. It should be recognised, however, that in old age, epilepsy may not present with the full blown picture of an aura followed by convulsions. The patient may simply lose consciousness. If it seems likely that the patient has epilepsy, an attempt should be made to distinguish between that due to cerebrovascular disease and that resulting from a benign or malignant tumour. A careful history and examination accompanied by simple investigations such as a chest X-ray may give the answer. If doubt remains more sophisticated tests such as electroencephalography, isotope scanning or computerised axial tomography should be considered. Which tests are chosen is, to some extent, dependent on local availability and often a therapeutic trial of an anticonvulsant may give a quicker and more effective answer.

## Cardiovascular disease

Blackouts may also result from heart block or transient or continuous arrhythmias, while syncope preceded by dizziness often is the result of postural hypotension. These disorders are discussed in more detail in Chapter 10.

## Other neurological conditions

Most other common neurological conditions also occur in old age and in some cases they will have existed for a long time. These conditions include multiple sclerosis, subacute combined degeneration of the spinal cord, motor neurone disease, peripheral neuropathies and neurosyphilis. Their management is the same as in younger age groups but their course may be different, motor neurone disease for instance running a longer and less severe course. Neurosyphilis is very rare now, but positive serological tests are not uncommon in old people who have neurological signs. While this finding may be of little significance, suggesting a past but not inactive infection, treatment with a course of penicillin often improves well-being and performance. It should also be remembered that the need and desire for sexual intercourse does not necessarily decrease in old age and consequently sexually transmitted diseases may occur.

Neuralgia also occurs in the elderly. Post-herpetic neuralgia is the commonest form and can be very troublesome. Early diagnosis of herpes zoster and treatment with idoxuridine may be the most effective way of preventing neuralgia but other treatment, apart from appropriate analgesics, is disappointing, although physiotherapy using massage with a vibrator on the painful area may be effective. Trigeminal neuralgia is less common. It may respond to carbamazepine (Tegretol) but neurosurgical methods may be necessary in resistant cases.

## Further reading

Adams G F (1974) *Cerebrovascular Disability.* Edinburgh: Churchill Livingstone

Caird F I (1982) *Neurological Disorders in the Elderly.* Bristol: Wright

Calne D B & Eisler T (1979) The pathogenesis and medical treatment of extrapyramidal diseases. *Med Clin N Amer*, **63**, 715–727

Garroway W M, Akhtar A J, Hockey, L & Prescott R J (1980) Management of acute stroke in the elderly: follow-up of a controlled trial. *Br Med J*, **2**, 822–829

Harrison M J G & Wilson L A (1978) Prevention of stroke. *Br J Hosp Med,* **20**, 444–445

Johnstone M (1983) *Restoration of Motor Function in the Stroke Patient.* Edinburgh: Churchill Livingstone

Noltie K & Denham M J (1981) Subdural haematoma in the elderly. *Age and Ageing*, **10**, 241–246

Norris J W & Hanchinski V C (1982) Misdiagnosis of stroke. *Lancet*, **1**, 328–331

Prudham D & Grimley Evens J (1981) Factors associated with falls in the elderly: a community study. *Age & Ageing*, **10**, 141–146

Turnbull J C & Aitken J A (1983) Diagnosis and management of Parkinsonism in the elderly. *Age & Ageing*, **12**, 309–316

Wild D, Nayak U S L & Isaacs B (1981) How dangerous are falls in old people at home? *Br Med J*, **282**, 266–268

# CHAPTER 9

# Brain Failure

Young people have bigger brains than old people, but this may be simply because in childhood they enjoyed a better state of health and nutrition than their grandparents did 50 or 60 years ago.

The human nerve cell has such highly specialised function that it is unable to reproduce itself. This means that the longer a person lives the more likely are disease and dengeneration to result in the death of neurones, and thus a reduction in the total number of brain cells. The brains of old people contain many fewer neurones than those of young people. This finding should be interpreted with caution, however. Accompanying any reduction in the number of brain cells there is a generalised reduction in the concentrations of substances involved in nerve transmission within the cerebral cortex. These include noradrenaline, acetylcholine and gamma-amino-butyric acid. Various structural changes are also found on histological examination of the cerebral cortex. These include oval plaques of degenerative material between neurones (senile plaques) and tangles of dilated microtubules within neurones (neurofibrillary tangles).

Some old people undergo an accelerated loss of nerve cells resulting in atrophy of the cerebral cortex. Histological examination reveals high concentrations of senile plaques and neurofibrillary tangles, the numbers of which bear a direct relationship to the cognitive ability of an individual. At a biochemical level there is a gross reduction in enzyme activity specific to that related to acetycholine metabolism. The part of the brain most severely affected by these changes is the hippocampus, a structure intimately associated with memory processing and storage. There is debate as to whether the condition represents an accelerated form of ageing, or if it is a distinct disease entity. The specific changes in acetylcholine metabolism suggest the latter.

Comparison of young and old subjects suggest that, on average, old people have a lower intellectual capacity than their younger counterparts. The apparent effect of ageing here is exaggerated by the fact that, by and large, young people have been better nourished, have had less childhood illness and have had more educational opportunities than earlier generations. Even allowing for these differences, however, ageing would appear to have an effect on cognitive ability. The main area of difficulty is in processing new information. An old person may be able to repeat immediately a series of numbers, but will have difficulty in repeating them a few hours or days later. He has little difficulty in recalling information learnt many years previously, particularly where this information was of importance to him. Thus it is that old people have difficulty in learning new skills, but have less difficulty in performing tasks dependent on past experience.

### Brain failure

The subtle changes in mental function described above should not be confused with changes associated with an inability to cope with everyday tasks found in some old people. Such a change is indicative of a disease rather than an ageing process. This condition has been variously described as dementia or a senile psychosis. In this book the term 'brain failure' is used. The value of the term is that it categorises brain function in the same way as that used for many other organs. Thus, acute brain failure implies a sudden deterioration in cerebral function. As with acute renal failure, this often is due to malfunction in other systems such as those of the alimentary tract or heart and blood vessels. In chronic brain failure the impairment is long standing. Like chronic renal failure the condition may be subject to acute exacerbations and, again, like chronic renal failure, may have an underlying treatable cause.

### Prevalence

Though not the direct result of ageing, chronic brain failure is rare in youth and middle age. Over the age of 65 it shows an exponential rise in both men and women from less than 5 per cent in those between 65 and 69 to over 20 per cent in those over 80 (Fig. 9.1). Though the prevalence is similar for a given age in the two sexes, there are many more women than men with chronic brain failure. This is simply due to women, on average, living longer than men.

Only 20 per cent of people with moderate to severe brain failure have been identified as such by their general practitioners. The others may only emerge when a crisis such as a bereavement, or an illness in the family makes it apparent that an old person is no longer able to cope. Earlier identification would allow relatives and professionals to plan for the future so that later problems could be predicted and thus, minimised.

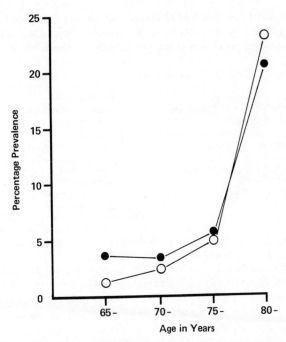

Figure 9.1   Prevalence of chronic brain failure in men ●
and women ○ (Wells 1979)

## Aetiology

About half of old people exhibiting signs and symptoms of chronic brain
failure are suffering from Alzheimer's disease, a condition characterised
by loss of brain cells and the presence of large numbers of senile plaques
and neurofibrillary tangles (see above). Some doctors restrict the term
Alzheimer's disease to patients under 65, describing the condition in
those over 65 as senile dementia. Since the histology and the clinical
presentation is similar whatever the age of the patient, the distinction
seems artificial, and the term Alzheimer's disease makes it clear that the
patient is suffering from an illness rather than from the effects of ageing.
Another approach is to describe the condition as being 'senile dementia
of the Alzheimer type' (SDAT).

A quarter of patients with chronic brain failure have multiple cerebral
infarcts, resulting from a high blood pressure, or from cerebral artery
stenosis and thrombosis due to atheroma. Here intellectual impairment is
due to a patchy destruction of brain tissue (multi-infarct dementia). The

condition occurs more often in men than women; tends to affect a slightly younger age group; and produces stepwise deterioration, unlike the relentless course found in Alzheimer's disease. It also is associated with

Table 9.1   Causes of Chronic Brain Failure

| | |
|---|---|
| Alzheimer's disease | Hypothyroidism |
| Multiple cerebral infarctions | Chronic renal failure |
| Cerebral tumour | Chronic liver failure |
| Chronic subdural haemorrhage | Parkinsonism |
| Recurrent trauma (boxing) | Recurrent hypoglycaemia |
| Alcoholism | Hypercalcaemia |
| Low pressure hydrocephalus | Hypokalaemia |
| Pick's disease | Neurosyphilis |
| Jakob–Creutzfeldt's disease | $B_{12}$, folic acid and nicotinic |
| Huntington's chorea | acid deficiency |

focal neurological abnormalities; produces patchy cognitive impairment; and often is accompanied by emotional lability.

Yet another sizeable group have Alzheimer's disease and multiple cerebral infarcts concurrently. The remainder suffer from one of the wide range of disorders listed in Table 9.1. Though small, this group is important since many of the disorders can be prevented, treated or even reversed.

A wide range of conditions may be responsible for the onset of acute brain failure (Table 9.2). These may cause a mental disturbance in any old person, but are even more likely to cause trouble if there is some degree of underlying chronic brain failure. Such patients often present with a complex mix of physical and psychiatric symptoms so that the combined skills of both physician and psychiatrist may be required. For this reason there is advantage in a geriatrician and a psychiatrist with an interest in the elderly combining forces in a joint psychiatric-geriatric assessment unit, where patients with acute brain failure can be assessed initially before transfer to whichever service ultimately proves to be more appropriate.

### Acute brain failure

In this condition there is some clouding of consciousness so that the doctor may have difficulty in attracting the attention of the patient, and even greater difficulty in sustaining an interest in the interview. Mental function tends to fluctuate so that it may be worse late in the day and immediately after waking. The patient has little control over emotions, and normally subconscious material. Thus, if normally anxious he may present with terror; if depressed may be suicidal; or suspicious may be paranoid. People and objects tend to be misidentified, and material normally presenting in dreams often surfaces as hallucinations.

Fundamental to the management of acute brain failure is identification

Table 9.2  Causes of Acute Brain Failure

| Infective | Electrolyte Imbalance |
|---|---|
| Bronchopneumonia | Dehydration |
| Pyelonephritis | Drugs, eg. diuretics |
| Local skin lesions | Renal failure |
| Diverticular abscess | Hypercalcaemia |
| Bacterial endocarditis | |
| | Endocrine |
| | Hypothyroidism |
| Neurological | Diabetes: hypoglycaemia |
| Drugs with a central | hyperglycaemia |
| neurological action | Hyperparathyroidism |
| Cerebral arteriosclerosis | |
| 'Stroke' | Nutritional |
| Cerebral tumour | 'Cachexia' |
| Subdural haematoma | $B_{12}$ deficiency |
| Epilepsy | Thiamine deficiency |
| | ? Folate deficiency |
| Cardio-respiratory | Miscellaneous |
| Myocardial infarction | Anaesthetic agents |
| Congestive cardiac failure | Trauma (surgical/accidental) |
| Pulmonary emboli | Tissue anoxia (gangrene) |
| Respiratory failure | Sudden isolation |
| Acute haemorrhage | Poisons, eg. digitalis |

of the underlying physical or mental disorder responsible (Table 9.2). The doctor's first difficulty is that information from the patient is likely to be unreliable. It is important, therefore, that he interviews people able to give a background to the crisis. These may include relatives, neighbours, a home help, a health visitor, a district nurse, a social worker and the general practitioner. These people often are more easily contacted at the patient's own home. It is also there that the doctor himself may pick up useful clues such as half consumed bottles of sherry, cupboards full of drugs, or grossly inadequate heating. A home assessment visit, preferably with the general practitioner may thus be extremely useful.

Treatment ultimately is dependent on identifying and treating the underlying cause, but while the medical staff are endeavouring to do this the nursing staff can do a great deal to minimise disruption and distress by a correct approach to the patient. Agitation is reduced if he can see what is going on and is not disturbed by a lot of background noise. He should be nursed, therefore, in a well-lit, but quiet room. Disorientation will be reduced if staff identify themselves, explain any procedures they are going to undertake, and frequently give information about time and surroundings. Visual hallucinations are more likely to occur in darkness so that at night a small light should be on in the room. Again sounds such as running water are liable to misinterpretation so that the patient should be well away from such distractions. If he seems to be living in the past, going through previous unpleasant experiences, it helps if his family can provide information on these so that staff can talk about them to the patient and provide him with reassurance.

The patient may resist attempts at medication or nursing procedures. Painstaking explanation helps to reduce this problem. Again it helps to appreciate that he sees many contacts as an unwarranted attack on his security and dignity. Finally, he may be irritable because he is in pain or discomfort. Relief of a faecal impaction or urinary retention, or treatment of a pressure area may solve the problem.

Tranquillisers may be required, but should be given in the correct dosage. Too small a dose will merely produce even more clouding of consciousness and increase agitation. Too large a dose may push the patient into coma increasing the risk of pressure sores and intercurrent chest infection. Oral preparations include chlorpromazine, thioridazine tablets or syrup, and haloperidol drops. Intramuscular injections may be necessary and, here, chlorpromazine, promazine or haloperidol may be used. In extreme cases prolonged sedation is required. This can be achieved with an intravenous infusion of chlormethiazole, but the rate has to be controlled by a pump, and the nursing staff have to keep a constant watch on the level of consciousness.

If the patient is restless at night, a hypnotic should be used, but if this is used it should be in a dose adequate to produce a sound sleep. It otherwise may leave him in a limbo of nightmares and hallucinations. The duration of action should also be short so that he is not left in a state of drowsiness the following day. Chlormethiazole tablets or capsules fulfil these criteria, as do short acting benzodiazepines such as temazepam. Barbiturates and long acting benzodiazepines such as nitrazepam should be avoided in this situation.

## Chronic brain failure

One of the earliest features of chronic brain failure is a poor memory for recent events. This often is accompanied by disabilities in abstract thinking, judgement and self-criticism. In their early stages these changes may be indistinguishable from variants of normality, so that it often is relatives rather than professionals who first identify the alteration in cognitive function and personality.

As the condition progresses forgetfulness becomes more serious so that instead of merely forgetting names the patient may forget to switch off a cooker, or go out into the street adequately dressed. At this stage variations in personality become accentuated so that a forthright person may become rude, a forceful individual aggressive and a timid patient tearful and agitated. In some instances, a strong personality may serve to disguise underlying impairment. Thus, a gregarious old lady will continue to chat cheerfully to her friends, and it may be some time before they realise that she is talking complete nonsense. If unable to give the right answer she obligingly makes one up (confabulates). Thus, an arthritic old lady in a long stay ward may say that she has been out shopping all morning, and that she has come home to cook her mother's lunch.

At a later stage of the disease there are serious changes in behaviour. The patient dresses untidily, eats sloppily, and gives up any attempt to cook or do housework. She may urinate and defaecate in the wrong places or simply become incontinent of urine and faeces. Wandering often is a problem, in that the patient may visit neighbours or go shopping in the middle of the night, and then forget why she has come out or where she has come from.

At the final stages, extensive cerebral damage results in the patient developing muscle weakness, spasticity, ataxia, and flexion contractures. She lies permanently curled up in bed, her only response to stimuli being to grasp or suck objects. Mercifully the patient then develops a bronchopneumonia and dies.

There is considerable variation in the rate at which patients with chronic brain failure deteriorate. Some old people do not progress beyond a mild degree of forgetfulness, and there is debate as to whether this represents a normal variant of ageing, or a 'benign' form of chronic brain failure. Whatever the explanation, the practical point at issue is that a doctor should not issue a gloomy prognosis on the basis of simple forgetfulness. He should, however, identify the patient as being at risk and arrange for him to be kept under regular review.

**Diagnosis.** A diagnosis of chronic brain failure can usually be made by taking a careful history from relatives and, sometimes, neighbours. In assessing prognosis, and planning support, however, it is useful to attempt to quantify the severity of the impairment. Aspects covered include orientation for time, place and people, memory for recent events, memory for distance events, and numeracy. This can be done using a simple questionnaire (Table 9.3). The test has its limitations. Deaf or dysphasic patients score badly; the patient may think the questions are silly; and depression or acute brain failure rather than chronic brain failure may be responsible for a poor score. Finally, a patient recently

Table 9.3   Mental Test Questionnaire

Name .......................................... Date ..............

|  | Score |
|---|---|
| Name | 0/1 |
| Age | 0/1 |
| Time (to nearest hour) | 0/1 |
| Time of day | 0/1 |
| Name and address for 5 minute recall: this should be repeated by the patient to ensure that it has been heard correctly: | |
| Mr John Brown | 0/1/2 |
| 42 West Street | 0/1/2 |
| Southsea | 0/1 |
| Day of week | 0/1 |
| Date (correct day of month) | 0/1 |
| Month | 0/1 |
| Year | 0/1 |
| Place: Type of place (ie. hospital) | 0/1 |
| Name of hospital | 0/1 |
| Name of ward | 0/1 |
| Name of town | 0/1 |
| Recognition of two persons (doctor, nurse, etc.) | 0/1/2 |
| Date of birth (day and month sufficient) | 0/1 |
| Place of birth (town) | 0/1 |
| School attended | 0/1 |
| Former occupation | 0/1 |
| Name of wife, sib., or next of kin | 0/1 |
| Date of World War I (year sufficient) | 0/1 |
| Date of World War II (year sufficient) | 0/1 |
| Name of present Monarch | 0/1 |
| Name of Prime Minister | 0/1 |
| Months of year backwards | 0/1/2 |
| Count 1–20 | 0/1/2 |
| Count 20–1 | 0/1/2 |
| Total | __ |

admitted to hospital tends to be flustered, and often performs badly. It is useful to wait three or four days until he has settled before giving the test. Accepting these limitations, a score of over 25 means that an individual may continue to manage to live independently; between 15 and 24 independent living is unlikely; and under 15 institutional care will be necessary unless there is considerable support in the home.

Another important dimension of chronic brain failure is behaviour. In assessing this, ward staff are asked to score performance in a spectrum of tasks in grades ranging from 0 to 5. This system is useful in providing both a pattern, and overall score for behavioural abnormality.

**Management.**  *Drug treatment.*  In Alzheimer's disease or after multiple cerebral infarctions, there are no drugs which produce a substantial improvement in mental function. Cerebral vasodilators should be avoided since they tend to dilate healthy vessels, and shunt blood away from ischaemic areas of the brain. A variety of agents modify cerebral metabolism, but though they sometimes produce a marginal improvement in cognitive ability, this rarely is sufficient to make a practical difference to the patient. An area of topical interest is an investigation into ways to correct abnormalities of acetylcholine metabolism found in Alzheimer's disease (see above). As yet, however, there is no evidence that treatment with the acetylcholine precursors choline, lecithin or deanol is of clinical benefit.

Treatment with a phenothiazine such as thioridazine or chlorpromazine may be useful if a patient is agitated or is inclined to wander. Care should be taken not to undersedate him so that he merely becomes disinhibited and even more restless; or oversedated so that he tends to sleep most of the time, has frequent falls and goes off his legs. A hypnotic such as chlormethiazole may be useful in controlling nocturnal restlessness, but here again, care should be taken to avoid excessive drowsiness the next morning. Chronic brain failure often is accompanied by depression, and the judicious use of antidepressants in appropriate cases may be helpful.

*Social support.*  Eighty per cent of patients with chronic brain failure live in their own homes, and places in residential homes and mental hospitals are heavily oversubscribed. It is essential, if health and social services are to continue to function, that resources be directed to keeping as many of these people at home as possible, by giving adequate support to their families. Help may consist of giving advice on applying for an attendance allowance, providing a laundry service for incontinence, or providing relief with regular visits to a day centre (Chapter 4). A community psychogeriatric nurse may perform regular visits to give reassurance and advice, and to report back to the psychiatric service.

In some parts of the country, self-help groups of relatives have been formed, often at the instigation of a psychiatrist or social worker. Regular meetings of these can do a great deal in relieving the tensions and worries involved in looking after a mentally frail relative.

If, despite this support, the family continue to be under a strain, attendance at a psychogeriatric day hospital may be prescribed. The unit ideally should be staffed by doctors and nurses, and other professionals such as an occupational therapist, clinical psychologist, speech therapist, social worker or teacher. Its primary aim is to maximise the self-care capacity of the patient. Specific techniques include the use of word and colour cues in improving memory; discussing everyday events to improve orientation; using the speech therapist to tackle communication problems, matching activities to the previous personality of the patient; managing behavioural problems with modification techniques; and helping the patient to structure his day. Other rôles of the day hospital are to assess suitability for a residential home or care at a day centre; to maintain performance at its baseline level; and to relieve social pressures on the family.

A family is more likely to keep a patient at home if it knows that when a crisis arises, the hospital will be able to respond immediately. The psychogeriatric unit should thus keep places for acute admissions. It should also keep places for regular short term relief admission, and thus stave off the time when long term hospital care becomes necessary.

Unfortunately, a rising proportion of old patients with mental impairment find themselves without family support. Here back up from social work departments, or sheltered housing may contain the situation. Particular attention may have to be given to problems such as wandering, or leaving gas taps on. These often can be tackled if they are clearly defined (Chapter 2); for example, fitting a double lock to the front and back door will keep a patient within the protected environment of his house, and fail safe gas taps can be fitted. Even with these, however, long term admission is usually necessary at an earlier stage than in patients with families.

## Long-term care

Obviously, in spite of the attempt to maintain patients in the community, the time may come when institutional care is required. This, like all other aspects of care of patients with chronic brain failure, should be pre-planned. Ideally, placement in residential accommodation should be attempted and the establishment of so-called 'special' residential homes may be justified. Here patients with mild or moderate chronic brain failure often accompanied by considerable physical disability can be housed within the local community (Homes for the Elderly Mentally Infirm). When such places have adequate medical supervision and support either from hospital specialists or from interested general practitioners, a good environment can be engendered which, in turn, has a favourable effect on staff morale and recruitment. In such institutions, classical custodial care régimes should be abandoned and attempts made to encourage residents to maintain as independent a rôle for the activities of daily living as is compatible with their condition. The more this is developed the more surprising it is how patients can and do respond to a positive approach. This has obvious benefits for both patients and staff.

The appropriate placement of patients with chronic brain failure in local authority homes and in psychiatric or geriatric departments depends not only on the degree of their behavioural disturbance and physical disability but also on the tolerance and training of the caring staff. Further, whether patients should be maintained altogether in one ward or wing or scattered throughout different areas is a question which must be answered in the light of local circumstances. A clear policy, however, must be agreed and followed so that admission of the elderly patient with chronic brain failure is not denied. The provision of an adequate psychogeriatric service involving both the hospital and the community goes far to avoid these conflicts, with resulting benefits to patients and a greater efficiency in the use of hospital beds.

The objective of long-term hospital care for patients with chronic brain failure should be similar. To this end patients should be constantly encouraged to feed themselves at the table, and mobility, even with its attendant risks, should be encouraged. The physical environment should either be adapted or purpose-built with these aims in mind. A large well-lit and well-decorated day room is mandatory. Vivid door colours should be used for identifying toilet areas; similarly, bed coverings should be coloured to enable the patients to find their own beds. The whole atmosphere of the patient's day should be focused towards activity. For these reasons a high staff/patient ratio is required, although not all the staff need to be professionals. Voluntary workers or relatives should be encouraged to participate in the patients' activities and to suggest activities of their own. Relatives should be consulted to determine the various pre-morbid preferences of the patients. Not all patients enjoy playing bingo, watching television or joining in sing-songs, and individual preferences should be catered for. In order to attempt to orientate the patients to the passage of time, frequent trips outside the ward will allow many to appreciate the changing seasons; raised gardens that the patients work themselves are extremely useful in this respect. Other activities include painting, soft toy making and singing. The activities, and there are many others, do not require highly skilled professional staff

– positive attitudes are far more important. Many units of this nature find local school children and students are most willing to help, and the patients themselves seem to relate extremely well to the younger age groups.

## Further reading

Arie T (1983) Pseudodementia. *Br Med J*, **286**, 1301–1302

Deakin J F W (1983) Alzheimer's disease: recent advances and future prospects. *Br Med J*, **287**, 1323–1324

Ford J M & Roth W T (1977) Do cognitive abilities decline with age. *Brit J Hosp Med*, **32**, 59–62

Levy R & Post F (1982) *The Psychiatry of Late Life*. Oxford: Blackwell Scientific Publications

McCormack D & Whitehead A (1981) The effect of providing recreational activities on the engagement level of long stay patients. *Age & Ageing*, **10**, 287–291

Pearce J & Miller E (1973) *Clinical Aspects of Dementia*. London: Baillière Tindall

Pitt B (1982) *Psychogeriatrics: An Introduction to the Psychiatry of Old Age*. Edinburgh: Churchill Livingstone

Roberts P J (ed) (1982) *The Biochemistry of Dementia*. Chichester: Wiley

Sheldon F (1982) Supporting the supporters: working with the relatives of patients with dementia. *Age & Ageing*, **11**, 184–188

Wells N E J (1979) *Dementia in Old Age*. London: Office of Health Economics

Whitehead J A (1979) *Psychiatric Disorders in Old Age*. Chichester: HM & M Publishers/Wiley

# CHAPTER 10

# The Cardiovascular System

## Pathology

Ageing is accompanied by a variety of changes in the heart and blood vessels. Thus, cells in heart muscle (myocardium) contain increasing concentrations of a brown pigment (lipofuscin). This represents a failure of the cells to clear themselves of waste products, and as yet its effect on cardiac function has been poorly defined. In between muscle fibres, an amorphous material with characteristic staining properties (amyloid) is deposited. As the process continues, heart muscle is squeezed out of existence so that in very old patients amyloid deposition is an important cause of heart failure. Ageing also is accompanied by the replacement of conduction tissues by fibrous tissue and this, in part, accounts for the high incidence of abnormal heart rhythms and blockage to heart conduction found in old age. Fibrous tissues in the heart valves may be replaced with soft gelatinous material (mucoviscoidosis) so that the valves malfunction. Again, fibrous rings around heart valves may become calcified. This also may interfere with valve function.

In larger blood vessels such as the aorta there is a change in the structure of connective tissue to that it becomes weaker and less elastic. This accounts for dilatation and elongation of these vessels. It also accounts, in part, for some of the changes in blood pressure described later.

## Physiology

All these changes have an important effect on cardiac function. Thus, the amount of blood the heart can push out at each beat (stroke volume) is reduced. The maximum rate at which the heart can beat also is reduced – at a given age the maximum pulse rate can be calculated roughly by subtracting the age in years from 220. Both these changes result in a diminution in the amount of blood the heart can pump out (cardiac output). At rest this does not create problems but under stress such as exercise it severely limits the activity of the subject. The effect of age on exercise should not be over-emphasised, however. A healthy man of 80 may not be able to run for a bus, but he should be able to walk up a hill or play a round of golf. If he cannot do this, he either is out of condition or is suffering from a disease.

## Coronary artery disease

Atheroma of the coronary arteries is a good example of a condition which is more common in old age but which does not fulfil criteria considered to be prerequisites of an ageing process (Table 10.1). The condition certainly

Table 10.1   Pre-requisites of an Ageing Process

| | |
|---|---|
| 1 | Should be an adverse effect |
| 2 | Should not be affected by external factors |
| 3 | Should occur in all members of a species |
| 4 | Should produce a steadily progressive change |

is harmful, but its incidence is affected by a wide range of external environmental factors (Table 10.2). Again it does not affect all groups of people equally being very much more common, for example, in Finns and Yugoslavians. Finally, rather than producing progressive deterioration, it usually is punctuated by episodes of acute illness often followed by gradual improvement until the next acute episode.

Table 10.2   Aetiological Factors in Arteriosclerosis

| | |
|---|---|
| Smoking | Obesity |
| Hypertension | High saturated fat diet |
| Lack of exercise | Familial hyperlipidaemia |
| Diabetes mellitus | Hypothyroidism |

One of the most common manifestations of coronary artery disease is chest pain (angina) on exertion. Though the condition causes a great deal of apprehension there is some room for optimism in that many patients with angina in middle age lose this in old age. Sometimes this is due to the patient simply taking less exercise. More usually it represents a real improvement brought about by the development of a collateral circulation. The mainstay of treatment is glyceryl trinitrate, a substance absorbed from the buccal mucosa. Unfortunately, it often produces unpleasant palpitations or a feeling of faintness. Drugs which reduce the work of the heart such as the beta-blocking agent propranolol are useful, but should be used with caution in old people since they can precipitate cardiac failure in susceptible individuals. Another useful drug is nifedipine. This reduces the utilisation of oxygen by the heart, and causes peripheral vasodilatation.

If an old person has persistent angina he may require extra support in the form of a home help, or even rehousing, if he lives at the top of a hill or up several flights of stairs. Sometimes in geriatric practice it is the spouse rather than the patient who has angina. This should be taken into account, and extra support laid on when considering the discharge of such a patient.

## Coronary thrombosis

In its classical presentation, coronary thrombosis produces a severe crushing chest pain lasting at least half an hour and radiating down the left arm or up into the jaw. This pattern often is absent in older patients. They may complain merely of breathlessness, palpitations, dizziness or generalised weakness, or may quite suddenly become confused and disorientated (Chapter 9). Explanations for the atypical presentation of coronary thrombosis in old age include an increased threshold for ischaemic pain, a reduced immunological response to infection or ischaemia, or a more stoical response to symptoms. Other old people with mental impairment may be unable to give a clear account of their symptoms. Whatever the explanation, the lesson is that if there is a sudden deterioration in the health of an elderly patient it is always worth considering the possibility of a coronary thrombosis.

An important principle in the management of coronary thrombosis in old age is that bed rest should be restricted to patients with complications such as hypotension, an arrhythmia or cardiac failure. In other circumstances, prolonged bed rest will almost certainly immobilise the patient and condemn him to a prolonged period of rehabilitation. Another disadvantage of bed rest is that it results in venous stasis increasing the risk of deep leg vein thrombosis, and subsequent embolism of a clot to the lung (Chapter 11). The danger is not eliminated entirely by sitting the patient in a chair. Gentle mobilisation as soon as the patient feels well enough should be encouraged.

Some patients with coronary thrombosis die during defaecation. The danger is reduced by giving a stool softening agent such as dioctyl sulphosuccinate; and using a commode rather than a bedpan. Trying to defaecate while balancing in bed on top of a bedpan is an extremely strenuous and hazardous business.

Coronary thrombosis often is an alarming illness, and anxiety is increased if the patient is admitted to a coronary care unit and attached to sophisticated monitoring equipment. Unless the patient is suffering from a complication of the disease, there is no evidence that such an approach has any effect on mortality and morbidity. In most circumstances the patient will be happier if he is managed in his own home. If this is done, however, the family must be given advice on managing such problems as constipation, and on the importance of early mobilisation. Regular visits by the general practitioner and district nurse also are essential in maintaining the morale of relatives. If the family are unable to cope because of disability or anxiety, or if the patient is living alone, he should be admitted to hospital. There is usually advantage in his going into a geriatric rather than an acute medical unit. Here the pace is slower and there is less noise and activity at night.

Once the patient has recovered steps should be taken to prevent recurrence. Even in old age advice on stopping smoking, taking regular exercise, reducing weight and controlling blood pressure are important. Anticoagulants are of no value in this situation. Again, there is no evidence that dipyridamole or sulphinpyrazone, agents that reduce platelet stickiness, work in this age group.

## Congestive cardiac failure

This is a condition in which an inadequate cardiac output results in the accumulation of excessive quantities of fluid on the venous side of the circulation (causes of failure are listed in Table 10.3). Manifestations of

Table 10.3   Causes of Cardiac Failure

| | |
|---|---|
| Hypertension | High output, eg. |
| Ischaemic heart disease | thiamine deficiency |
| Pulmonary disease | thyrotoxicosis |
| Senile amyloidosis | Paget's disease |
| Valvular disease | |

failure include fluid in the lungs and pleura, congestion of neck veins, oedema over the sacrum and ankles, and congestion and enlargement of the liver. In old people no single sign should be taken an indicating cardiac failure. Thus, jugular venous distension may be due to compression by a dilated subclavian artery; liver enlargement may be due to the spread of a tumour; and a few moist sounds often are heard at the bases of old people with a limited respiratory excursion. They usually disappear on coughing. One of the most difficult signs to interpret in old age is ankle oedema. There are many causes for this (Table 10.4). One of the more common of these in the geriatric unit is limited mobility. Old ladies who sit around all day are not using their leg muscles to pump blood up their leg veins to their abdomen and thorax. This eventually results in local oedema which tends to be resistant to treatment.

The mainstay in the treatment of congestive cardiac failure at present is diuresis. In the acute stages of the illness a rapidly acting diuretic such as frusemide or bumetanide may have to be used. Such agents have the

Table 10.4  Causes of Ankle Oedema

| | |
|---|---|
| Cardiac failure | Protein subnutrition |
| Hepatic cirrhosis | Chronic venous obstruction |
| Nephrotic syndrome | Immobility |

inevitable effect of causing severe frequency. In less mobile patients this results in incontinence. Treatment should therefore by changed as soon as possible for a longer acting thiazide diuretic. All diuretics can cause an imbalance of sodium, chloride or potassium so that in the initial stages of treatment these electrolytes should be closely monitored in the serum. Potassium depletion may be corrected by supplementation (Table 10.5) or prevented by using a potassium saving diuretic such as amiloride or triamterene. The danger of potassium retention must be remembered.

Digoxin and other cardiac glycosides help in cardiac failure by increasing the force of cardiac contraction. It also is useful in reducing the irregular tachycardia associated with atrial fibrillation. Unfortunately the drug has many serious side effects (Table 10.6). Its use should be restricted to patients with heart failure not responding adequately to diuretics, and to those with rapid atrial fibrillation. Another cause for caution in the use of digoxin for old people is that reduced renal function (Chapter 5) prolongs the already slow excretion of the drug. Old people, therefore, should be given a reduced loading dose of between 250 and 500 $\mu$g, and a maintenance one of 125 $\mu$g daily. In those with chronic renal failure, the maintenance dose may have to be reduced to 62.5 $\mu$g daily.

If ankle oedema is the result of stasis diuretics have little effect. A better approach is to encourage increased mobility while, at the same time, advising that the feet be elevated on a stool when the patient is resting.

Table 10.5  Potassium Supplements

| Preparation | Quantity of Potassium per Tablet/Sachet |
|---|---|
| Kloref tablets | 6–7 mmol |
| Kloref-S sachets | 20 mmol |
| Sando-K tablets | 12 mmol (but only 8 mmol Cl$^-$) |
| Slow K tablets | 8 mmol |

Table 10.6  Digoxin Side Effects

| | |
|---|---|
| Bradycardia | Confusion |
| Heart block | Gynaecomastia |
| Arrhythmias | Yellow vision |
| Nausea | |

Fluid also may be removed from the legs by tightly applying a one-way stretch 'blue line' bandage. Elastic stockings are of limited value in that they do not produce a sufficient force of compression. Another approach is to apply an alternating pressure air splint to the limb (Flotron, Boots).

## Abnormal rhythms

The most common abnormal rhythm in old age is atrial fibrillation. Causes include myocardial ischaemia, chronic rheumatic heart disease, thyrotoxicosis or respiratory infections. Digoxin is effective either by converting the heart back to sinus rhythm, or reducing the irregular heart rate to a level at which the efficiency of cardiac contraction is increased. If the atrial fibrillation is due to thyrotoxicosis or an infection, treatment of the underlying condition may make it possible to discontinue digoxin.

Other arrhythmias occurring in old people include sinus, supraventricular and ventricular tachycardias, and sinus bradycardia. Symptoms pointing to such lesions include palpitations, breathlessness, chest pain and dizziness. Often symptoms are atypical so that the patient merely may feel weak or may become confused. An electrocardiogram is essential in establishing the diagnosis. Supraventricular tachycardias may respond to digoxin, but ventricular ones are invariably treated by electrical cardioversion.

Old people with complete heart block may present with recurrent falls or blackouts. Equally they may feel tired or complain of failing memory. The pulse rate usually is 40 beats per minute or less. If the blockage is due to ischaemia the outlook is poor, but in old people it often is due to an age related fibrosis of the atrioventricular node. In this situation the outlook is excellent if the heart rate can be increased. This can be done by inserting a permanent battery operated pacemaker. There are few contra-indications to this procedure. Even patients with mental impairment may be improved once their heart rate is increased.

The diagnosis of an arrhythmia or heart block is easy if the patient is seen during an attack. Often, however, the episodes are intermittent and the patient or relatives give a story of recurrent falls, blackouts, transient focal neurological signs, or episodes of confusion. Here a careful history may distinguish from other causes of these symptoms (Chapter 8). Confirmation usually requires the use of a portable monitor to provide a 24-hour record of the heart rhythm. Most people and particularly old people have occasional abnormal beats, and these are of little relevance. For a transient arrhythmia to be important it must be associated with symptoms. During the recording, therefore, the patient may be asked to make a note of any untoward symptoms. Treatment is dependent on the arrhythmia identified, but in many instances the patient benefits from the insertion of a permanent pacemaker.

## Carotid sinus hypersensitivity

In young people, massage of the carotid sinus in the neck results in a slowing of the heart rate and a fall in blood pressure. Fortunately, the cerebral blood vessels rapidly adapt to these changes so that accidental compression of the sinus rarely causes symptoms. In old age, the carotid sinus usually is less sensitive to stimuli, but in the few patients in whom sensitivity is normal or enhanced, symptoms are common. The reason is that the cerebral arteries are rigid and thus adapt poorly to changes in blood flow. Thus a drop in pulse rate or fall in blood pressure is likely to cause faintness or even a loss of consciousness.

The diagnosis of carotid sinus hypersensitivity is made by massaging each carotid sinus, noting any change in heart rate on an electrocardiographic strip. In view of the risk of producing prolonged asystole the manoeuvre should only be performed where means of cardiac resuscitation are to hand. Once diagnosed, the condition responds well to sustained release isoprenaline, a beta-adrenergic receptor stimulator.

## Postural hypotension

When a healthy adult stands up from a lying or sitting position, a tendency for blood to pool in the legs is counteracted by an increased cardiac output, and constriction of small blood vessels in the legs. Any disturbance in this mechanism will result in a fall in blood pressure accompanied by a decrease in cerebral blood flow, so that the patient feels faint or may lose consciousness. Causes of this include a diminished

Table 10.7   Causes of Postural Hypotension

| | |
|---|---|
| (a) Damage to mid-brain or hypothamamus | Cerebrovascular disease |
| (b) Damage to autonomic nervous system | Parkinsonism |
| | Shy Drager syndrome |
| | Diabetes mellitus |
| (c) Reduced plasma volume | Dehydration |
| | Haemorrhage |
| (d) Potassium depletion | Diarrhoea |
| (e) Damaged peripheral blood vessels | Varicose veins |
| | Hypertension |
| (f) Autonomic nervous system disuse | Immobility |
| DRUGS | |
| (a) CNS suppressants | Barbiturates |
| | Benzodiazepines |
| (b) Anticholinergic agents | Tricyclic antidepressants |
| | Anti-Parkinsonian agents |
| | Phenothiazine tranquillisers |
| | Drugs used in incontinence |
| (c) Drugs causing fluid depletion | Diuretics |

blood volume due to diuretics, dehydration or haemorrhage. In other patients the autonomic nervous system regulating blood pressure may be damaged by ageing, disease, or drugs (Table 10.7).

Treatment of postural hypotension may consist simply of discontinuing an offending drug. Where the patient has been immobile for a long time, it may be necessary to exercise the autonomic nervous system. This can be done using a special table to alternate the patient between an erect and supine posture. More simply, he can be encouraged to take as many opportunities as possible to get on to his feet. If this does not work the volume of blood in the legs may be reduced by applying one-way stretch bandages or even using a pilot's pressure suit. Although interesting, this approach rarely is practical in most patients requiring geriatric care. If the patient is sufficiently cooperative, he also may be trained in isometric leg exercises designed to increase the flow of blood from his legs.

Drugs have also been used to treat the condition. An example is that the salt retaining corticosteroid fludrocortisone has been given to increase the blood volume. Unfortunately, it is often difficult to maintain a balance between control of blood pressure and overt fluid retention associated with signs of congestive cardiac failure. Drugs which merely stimulate the sympathetic nervous system are useless, but there is evidence to suggest that pindolol, a drug which paradoxically combines blockade of beta adrenergic receptors with increased sympathetic drive may be effective. Further work is required to establish whether or not the drug is a practical possibility in older patients.

## Valvular heart disease

Diseases of the aortic and mitral valves are common in old people. The most common causes are chronic rheumatic disease and various degenerative processes (Table 10.8). Ausculation of a cardiac murmur usually identifies the condition, but the severity of the lesion bears little relationship to the loudness of the murmur. A loud systolic murmur over the aortic valve may be due simply to some roughening of the valve cusps (aortic sclerosis). This will not have any appreciable effect on heart func-

Table 10.8   Causes of Valvular Disease

| Aortic valve | Mitral valve |
| --- | --- |
| Bicuspid valve | Rheumatic disease |
| Rheumatic disease | Calcification |
| Syphilis | Mucoviscoidosis |
| Aortic dilatation | Ruptured papillary muscles |
| Bacterial endocarditis | Bacterial endocarditis |

tion. A faint diastolic murmur heard over the mitral valve may be due to severe narrowing of the mitral valve. Some old people by virtue of chronic brain failure or generalised arterial disease are unfit for cardiac surgery and should be treated with diuretics or digoxin. Age itself, however, is not a barrier to surgery. Old people who are otherwise fit, show a low operative mortality and an excellent long term response to valvular surgery.

## Infections of the heart

Patients with damaged heart valves are at increased risk from endocardial infection. This can be precipitated by such procedures as a dental extraction, catheterisation of the urinary bladder or prostatectomy. Prior treatment with antibiotics will diminish the risk in susceptible individuals.

Table 10.9  Clinical Features of Bacterial Endocarditis

| | |
|---|---|
| Fever | Weight loss |
| Anaemia | Clubbing of fingers |
| Rapid pulse | Liver enlargement |
| Confusional state | Spleen enlargement |
| Heart failure not responding | Blood in urine |
| to treatment | Osler's nodes |

Table 10.9 lists the classical signs of the disease. These often are absent in old people who may present by feeling vaguely unwell, by having had a fall or by being mildly confused. A high index of suspicion is necessary if the condition is not to be missed. The diagnosis usually is suspected when a patient with valvular disease has a high ESR, and is confirmed by demonstrating an infected sample of blood. Repeated blood cultures may be required to do this. Treatment consists of giving large doses of the appropriate antibiotic. Even with this, there is a very high mortality.

## Hypertension

Many healthy old people have high blood pressures. This led many doctors to conclude that, in old age, the condition should be left untreated. More recently studies of large numbers of subjects over many years have established that, even in old age, a high blood pressure is associated with a greatly increased risk of both coronary thrombosis and cerebrovascular disease. It would appear that, contrary to popular opinion, a high systolic pressure may be just as important or even more important than a high diastolic one. Studies have at last confirmed that treating hypertension in the elderly reduces morbidity and mortality.

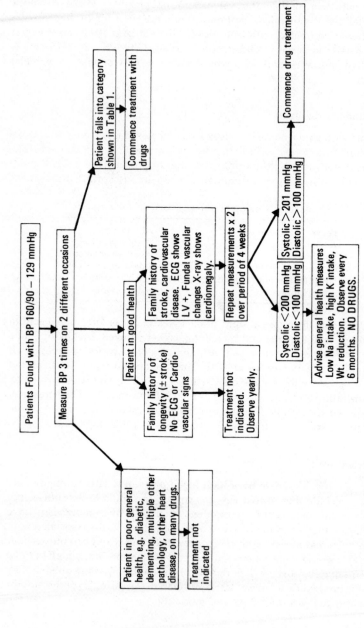

Figure 10.1 Flow chart to rationalise the management of hypertension in the elderly

The World Health Organisation defines hypertension as a blood pressure of more than 160/95. So many elderly people have blood pressures close to this level that it is probably wise to define a higher level before beginning treatment except in the younger elderly. However, there now is evidence that even over the age of 75 treatment of hypertension is beneficial. The indications for treatment are listed in Table 10.10 and a

Table 10.10   Indications for Treatment

1   Patients under 75 years already on
    hypotensive therapy
2   Patients with accelerated hypertension
3   Patients aged 60–69 with a BP >160/95
4   Patients aged 70–75 with a BP >180/100
5   Patients of any age with symptoms or
    with a previous stroke

flow chart to rationalise the management of hypertension in the elderly in Figure 10.1.

It must be remembered that general health measures such as weight reduction, exercise and diet may be as useful as drug therapy. If it is decided to use drugs then it is wise to introduce them in a step-like manner (Fig. 10.2). Which drug to use is the choice of the treating doctor –

Step 1:
Oral Diuretic                          — Hydrochlorothiazide

Step 2:
Addition of an adrenergic inhibitor
Beta adrenergic blockers — Propranolol
Alpha 2 agonists          — Methyl dopa — clonidine
Alpha 1 blocker           — Prazosin

Step 3:
Addition of a vasodilator,
Hydralazine (or Prazosin)

Figure 10.2   A stepped care approach to medical
treatment

commonly a thiazide diuretic or a beta-adrenoceptor blocking agent is used first and the other added to it if the first is ineffective. Alternative first choices may be nifedepine or verapamil. It must be remembered that all drugs produce hypostatic hypotension so that dizziness and falls may occur. Thiazides may cause urinary incontinence while the beta-adrenoceptor drugs may provoke heart failure and interact with verapamil and nifedepine.

If a third drug proves necessary, hydralazine or other vasodilator drugs may be used, but it is probably best to avoid the more potent adrenergic neurone-blocking drugs, and the centrally-acting hypotensive drugs, such as methyl dopa or clonidine.

## Peripheral arteries

Many old people suffer blockage to the arteries of their legs by athero-sclerosis. The condition may present initially as calf pain on exercise (claudication) or as pain in the skin of the foot when the limb is elevated and at rest. Progress of the condition can often be delayed by control of the precipitating factors, particularly smoking and diabetes mellitus (Table 10.2). The health visitor can educate and advise concerning these and other issues such as avoiding extremes of temperature, avoiding crowds where a crush injury may occur, and consulting a chiropodist rather than undertaking a 'do it yourself' foot surgery. All too readily a local foot infection is the episode which converts an 'at risk' foot into an acute emergency.

## Drugs and surgery

A wide range of drugs designed to dilate blood vessels or reduce blood viscosity have been used in peripheral arterial disease. There is little evidence that these are effective and their use should be resisted. Surgery involving the removal of an atheromatous plaque (endarterectomy), or by-passing the stenosed area with a Teflon graft or venous homograft, has much more to offer the patient. Here, limitations may be that atheroma is widespread in the arteries distal to the site of surgery, or that severe myocardial or cerebral atheromatous disease may prevent the patient from benefiting from peripheral vascular surgery.

## Amputation

If a large artery is completely blocked, rapid surgical intervention is necessary if the limb is to be saved. If delay occurs amputation is inevit-able. Here steps should be taken to ensure that the patient is in the fittest possible condition and is mentally and physically prepared for life with-out a limb. The decision to amputate should be taken early rather than late and the site of operation should be high enough to ensure a well-healed stump as soon as possible after the operation. If possible, the patient should be measured for a temporary pylon before operation, so that intensive physiotherapy using the prosthesis may begin immediately. If patients are considered unlikely to regain independence after amputation a decision should be taken to make them wheelchair independent. The prognosis for recovery to independence with a prosthesis or wheelchair is directly related to the enthusiasm and skill of the whole team undertaking rehabilitation (*see* Chapter 8).

## Further reading

Caird F I, Dall J L C & Kennedy R D (1976) *Cardiology in Old Age*. New York & London: Plenum Press

Hall M R P & Briggs R S J (1983) *Hypertension – A suitable case for treatment*. Geriatric Medicine, **13**, 685–690

Joint Working Party of the Royal College of Physicians of London and the British Cardiac Society (1976) Prevention of coronary heart disease. *J R Coll Physicians Lond*, **10**, 214–275

Martin A & Camm A J (1984) *Heart Disease in the Elderly*. Chichester: Wiley

Moulsdale M T, Eykyn S J & Phillips I (1980) Infective endocarditis, 1970–79. *Quart J Med*, **49**, 315–328

Pomerance A (1974) Pathology of heart disease in the elderly. *Br J Hosp Med*, **11**, 245–252

Wollner L (1978) Postural hypotension in the elderly. *Age & Ageing*, **7**(S), 112–118

# CHAPTER 11

# The Ageing Lung

## Ageing and ventilation

In healthy young people the levels of oxygen and carbon dioxide in arterial blood are kept within very narrow limits. Any fall in oxygen or rise in carbon dioxide results in a rapid increase in the depth and rate of respiration. In old age, degenerative changes of the ventilatory centres in the brain stem, and of the oxygen receptors in the carotid and aortic bodies, result in a diminished response to changes in these gases.

With increased age there is wasting of muscles in the diaphragm and intercostal spaces accompanied by calcification of costal cartilage, and degeneration of joints articulating ribs with the dorsal vertebrae. Compounding these changes in the thoracic cage the structure of connective tissue within the lung is modified so that collagen is replaced by pseudoelastin, a substance with a very low tensile stress. Thus it is that bronchioles become floppy and tend to collapse on expiration. The alveoli also are less elastic so that an increased force is required to empty them.

The physiological consequences of these changes are that when old people breath out they exert a decreased force on airways which are more prone to collapse, and alveoli which are more resistant to compression. The effect of this on the lung function tests is illustrated in Table 11.1, and Figure 11.1.

Table 11.1   Age Changes in Lung Function

| Static volumes: | Total lung capacity (TLC) | Unchanged |
|---|---|---|
| | Vital capacity | Decrease |
| | Functional residual capacity | Increase |
| | Residual volume | Increase |
| Dynamic volumes: | Forced expiratory volume (FEV) | Decrease |
| | Maximum breathing capacity | Decrease |
| | Peak expiratory flow | Decrease |

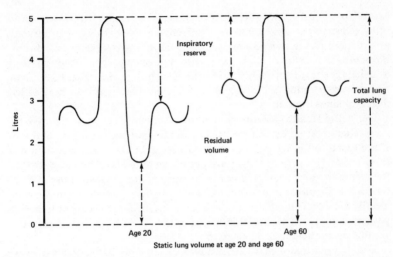

Figure 11.1   Static lung volume at age 20 and age 60

## Practical consequences

A reduced response to anoxia or hypercapnia (high carbon dioxide level) means that under conditions of stress such as a chest infection old people are more likely to develop a blood gas imbalance associated with drowsiness and confusion. The reduced efficiency of the thoracic cage and lungs means that old people tend to become more breathless with less exertion than young people; that there is a diminished respiratory excursion so that breath sounds are softer and abnormal sounds more difficult to detect when there is lung disease; and that the efficiency of coughing is impaired so that old people tend to accumulate bronchial secretion particularly when they are recumbent. There is the further problem that if lung function tests are performed in an elderly patient their pattern may mimic that found in obstructive airways disease in a younger patient. It is very important, therefore, that in interpreting lung function test the age of the patient should be taken into account.

## Obstructive syndromes

The three major obstructive syndromes are chronic bronchitis, emphysema and asthma. *Simple chronic bronchitis* is defined by the British Medical Research Council as an increase in the volume of mucoid bronchial secretions sufficient to cause expectoration on most days during three consecutive months for more than two successive years, with the exclusion of focal causes such as bronchiectasis. *Complicated chronic bronchitis* refers to the development of infective exacerbations or of airways obstruction giving rise to shortness of breath. The prevalence of chronic bronchitis as defined, increases with increasing age, although it is unusual for chronic bronchitis to begin over the age of 60 (Fig. 11.2). As in all other age groups, women are less affected than men; this may reflect different smoking habits.

The World Health Organisation defines *emphysema* as a condition of the lungs characterised by an increase beyond the normal in the size of the air space distal to the terminal bronchioles brought about by destruction of their walls. The patient with pure emphysema tends to be younger than the one with more classical chronic bronchitis, but because of the difficulties in the diagnosis of emphysema the figures for prevalence in the community are very difficult to obtain. Characteristically, the emphysematous patient complains of breathlessness, often at rest, in the absence of significant bronchial hypersecretion.

*Asthma* is a disease characterised by a variable resistance in the airways which may disappear either spontaneously or as a result of treatment. It used to be thought that asthma was a disease primarily of young people but increasingly it is being recognised in the elderly; indeed, it may arise for the first time in the extremely old. Unfortunately, it seems that the elderly are more likely to develop infective complications with asthma,

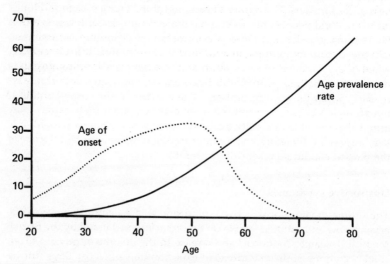

Figure 11.2   Chronic bronchitis in males (Fry 1966)

which makes it difficult to distinguish from chronic bronchitis with airways obstruction.

## Management of chronic obstructive syndromes

Every effort should be made to stop chronic bronchitic patients from smoking. This will not influence the progressive downhill nature of the disease, but will reduce the liability to recurrent infections, which when they occur, should be treated with a broad spectrum antibiotic. Doxycycline (Vibramycin) is probably the drug of choice for the elderly because of the ease of its once daily administration and the added advantage that it does not lead to an increase in the blood urea.

## Bronchodilators

Selective beta$_2$-adrenoceptor stimulants (sympathomimetics) such as salbutamol or terbutaline are of obvious benefit where there is bronchospasm. They are safe and effective and may be given as aerosol inhalations, as well as by mouth in most cases or parenterally in severe acute asthma. Some elderly find aerosols difficult to use and all patients should be taught how to use these. The mode of use should be demonstrated by patients at regular intervals as proof of its correctness. Those elderly who are unable to use aerosols may be prescribed dry powder inhalations – (Ventolin Rotacaps). Other modifications to inhalation include the 'spacer' and the 'Nebuhaler' both used with terbutaline (Bricanyl).

Non-selective adrenoceptor stimulants such as ephedrine may be used but are likely to cause cardiac irregularities. The xanthine derivatives, aminophylline and theophylline, if given as sustained release preparations may be useful. In this form they produce fewer adverse reactions and when given at night may control nocturnal wheezing. They may have a good prophylactic effect and can be used as an alternative to sodium cromoglycate.

Corticosteroids may sometimes need to be used to help control asthma. They should be used with caution in the elderly. Aerosol or dry powder inhalant forms are available and may be effective if used in conjunction with a selective beta$_2$-adrenoceptor stimulant. A home nebuliser may be necessary in those patients who cannot manage aerosol or dry powder inhalation.

Antihistamines may be used if hay fever or vasomotor rhinitis is troublesome. The newer antihistamines, such as astemizole, may be best used as it hardly penetrates the blood brain-barrier, causes fewer adverse reactions and has a once daily dosage.

There has been considerable debate about the use of oxygen in chronic obstructive airways disease. The most effective method would appear to be giving oxygen in a low concentration (25% oxygen) throughout 24 hours. The cost of the technique is such that it is not yet available for routine use in the patient's own home.

Table 11.2   Conditions Associated with Restrictive Syndromes

| | |
|---|---|
| Left ventricular failure | Fibrosing alveolitis |
| Rheumatoid lung | Drugs |
| Sarcoidosis | Ankylosing spondylosis |
| Systemic lupus | Severe kyphoscoliosis |
| Lupus erythematosis | |

## Restrictive syndromes

This term covers a number of syndromes with a characteristic ventilatory function pattern (Table 11.2). The vital capacity is markedly reduced, but measures of airways obstruction are relatively normal. The patient usually complains of breathlessness on exertion rather than at rest, and although extremely dyspnoeic is quite pink in colour. The production of sputum in these syndromes is unusual. A great number of diseases are known now to produce restrictive syndromes, but in the elderly left ventricular failure in both sexes and rheumatoid disease in females will account for the majority. Patients with restrictive syndromes do not usually retain carbon dioxide to any great extent except terminally, so domiciliary oxygen given intermittently is safe and may give considerable symptomatic relief. Bronchodilators usually are inappropriate.

## Pneumonia

Pneumonia is a common and often terminal event in old people. Reasons for this include an impaired cough mechanism, impaired local immunological defences, and the frequent association of diseases predisposing to respiratory infection such as cardiac or renal failure. Diagnosis often is difficult because the usual signs such as cough, sputum, fever and chest pain may be absent. Non-specific features such as falls, cardiac failure, confusion or reduced mobility are common. A raised respiratory rate of 28/min or more may be the most useful indication preceding physical signs or radiological change by as much as 48 hours.

Some gravely ill old people exhibit only minimal radiological changes. Sputum cultures are useful in identifying the guilty organisms. If the patient is uncooperative or unable to cough, a blood culture may be a useful alternative. Some elderly patients suffer from recurrent bouts of bronchopneumonia. Table 11.3 lists some of the causes. Chest X-rays may be useful in defining these and monitoring change.

Table 11.3  Causes of Recurrent Pneumonia

Obstruction: carcinoma
             foreign body
Pulmonary abscess
Tuberculosis
Repeated aspiration: debility
                     bed rest/recumbency
                     post-anaesthetic
                     oesophageal lesion
                     alcoholism

Although many causes of pneumonia in the elderly are treated adequately and successfully at home, many patients will undoubtedly benefit from skilled nursing which can be constantly available within the hospital. A suitable broad spectrum bactericidal antibiotic should be chosen. Unfortunately, it is not usually expedient to await the results of sputum and/or blood cultures, although it is often wise to obtain the specimens prior to antibiotic therapy so that this can be changed later in the light of bacterial sensitivity. Persistent or recurrent pneumonia always requires bacteriological investigation. Anoxia can be treated with oxygen therapy; if there is any evidence of pre-existing long-standing lung disease this should be of low concentration, ie. 28 per cent as provided by the Ventimask. Dehydration should preferably be prevented though this is often difficult as these ill patients are very reluctant to drink. If necessary, intravenous fluids should be administered, but great care must be taken to ensure that congestive cardiac failure and parotitis do not occur, as both may be precipitated by pneumonia, and require appropriate treatment.

**Tuberculosis**

While modern anti-tuberculous drugs have reduced the incidence of tuberculosis in the population at large, the condition remains relatively common in old people. Reasons for this are that they often have contracted the infection fifty or more years previously, and that diminished immunological defences accompanying ageing and ill health may allow a lung quiescent lesion to break down and become reactivated.

Tuberculosis may present with feverishness, night sweats, weight loss, a cough or haemoptysis. More often, in old age, the patient merely feels vaguely unwell. This can all too readily be attributed wrongly to ageing or depression.

The diagnosis of pulmonary tuberculosis can be made by identifying characteristic changes on the chest X-ray. Doubt often remains as to whether the changes are due to quiescent disease. The sputum should thus be examined under the microscope to identify tubercule bacilli, and a specimen sent off for guinea pig culture. If the patient is unwilling or unable to cough, a laryngeal swab often will provide appropriate material. A further approach is to perform a Mantoux test. Unfortunately, immunological changes often mean that even with active tuberculosis a skin test using a tuberculin concentration of 1/10,000 may be negative. Where this happens repeating the test with a 1/1,000 concentration usually will produce a skin response. If despite this the reaction is negative, a tuberculous infection is most unlikely. A positive reaction means that the patient either has active tuberculosis or has had it in the past.

The treatment currently recommended for tuberculosis in old age is to start with a combination of isoniazid, rifampicin and ethambutal (Table 11.4). If cultures establish that the infecting organism is sensitive to all three preparations, it is possible to continue maintenance treatment with isoniazid and rifampicin alone. Streptomycin and para-amino salicyclic acid are available for use where there is resistance or side effects to the other drugs. Usually, however, these two agents are more toxic than the others, and are best avoided initially.

Practical problems in the management of tuberculosis in old age is that it may persist unrecognised for years. This carries the risk to other members of the household (particularly children) getting infected and that the disease may have reached a very advanced stage before it is detected in the patient himself. A chest X-ray is mandatory, therefore, if there is the slightest possibility of there being tuberculosis. This is particularly important if the patient is going into an old people's home or a hospital. There also may be problems of drug compliance. Inadequate medication results not only in progression of the disease, but the development of resistant organisms. The doctor, health visitor or district nurse should keep a close watch on drug intake if this is to be avoided.

Table 11.4   Anti-tuberculous Drugs

|  | Max. Daily Dose |
|---|---|
| Rifampicin | 600 mg |
| Isoniazid | 300 mg |
| Ethambutol | 900 mg |
| Streptomycin | 500 mg |
| PAS | 12 g |

### Malignant disease

Lung cancer has a peak incidence in the over-70s. Pathologically, over half are squamous cell, approximately 30 per cent are anaplastic (including oat-cell) and the remainder are alveolar cell or adenocarcinomas. The presenting symptoms are often due to the effects of distant metastases. Persistent or recurrent pneumonia, dyspnoea, general malaise and weight loss are common, but unfortunately many of these symptoms are regarded as an inevitable consequence of growing old and are, therefore, disregarded by the patient and sometimes by his doctor. Haemoptysis and superior vena caval obstruction obviously point to the correct diagnosis, but non-metastatic neurological or endocrine syndromes may be the presenting features.

The objectives of investigation should be to establish the diagnosis, and to assess whether or not it is localised and thus amenable to curative treatment. Before embarking on expensive, dangerous and uncomfortable tests, it is important to consider whether or not the patient will be fit for active treatment. The lynch pin of diagnosis remains the plain chest X-ray depicting a mass, unilateral hilar enlargement, segmental collapse, a peripheral nodule, rib erosions or other radiological changes. If an expert cytologist is available, examination of the sputum for malignant cells will confirm the diagnosis in up to 80 per cent of cases. Bronchoscopy offers a direct view and local biopsy of the lesion, but only should be undertaken if surgery is contemplated. Other investigations such as tomography, pleural aspiration, pleural biopsy, and mediastinoscopy may be of value in particular patients.

Local resection of the tumour only stands a chance of being curative if there is rigorous selection of patients on the grounds of good general health, and absence of tumour spread. In other patients, radiotherapy should be considered, but only used where there are distressing complications such as haemoptysis, breathlessness, invasion of nerve plexuses, dysphagia or obstruction of the superior vena cava. If there are no symptoms, radiotherapy will merely make the patient feel ill, with no hope of permanent cure. The treatment of bronchial carcinoma with cytotoxic drugs or immunotherapy remains in its infancy and still is of unproven value.

The general management of malignant disease is dealt with in Chapter 15.

### Thrombo-embolic disease

Elderly patients are at increased risk of developing thrombosis in the deep veins of their calves and thighs. This results from venous stasis due to immobility or muscle weakness, venous congestion due to cardiac failure, and increased blood coagulability due to ischaemic and inflammatory conditions (Table 11.5).

Once it develops, the thrombosis may present with local tenderness,

Table 11.5   Peripheral Vein Thrombosis – Predisposing Factors

| | |
|---|---|
| Immobilisation | Obesity |
| Recumbancy | Hyperlipidaemia |
| Severe disease/disability | Varicose veins |
| Reduced cardiac output | Pelvic tumours |
| Fractures | (including faecal masses) |
| Malignant disease | Increased blood viscosity |

and lower limb oedema. The clinical signs often are minimal, however, and the first warning that something is wrong is when the patient sustains a pulmonary embolism in which a blood clot lodges in one of the pulmonary arteries. The classical symptoms of this include chest pain, breathlessness and haemoptysis. In old people these often are absent and the condition may present as acute brain failure (Chapter 9), a fall (Chapter 8), or generalised weakness. Examination of the chest may reveal diminished breath sounds and coarse crepitations over a lung segment, a pleural friction rub, or signs suggesting a pleural effusion; and a chest X-ray may show an area of lung collapse or a pleural effusion. These signs may be absent, in which case a definitive diagnosis only can be made by performing isotopic scans of the alveoli and of the pulmonary blood vessels. This will identify areas of arterial blockage.

Doctors and nursing staff should aim at preventing deep leg vein thrombosis. Old people are at increased risk of this if they are bedfast, or even if they are kept sitting in a chair all day. They should be encouraged to walk even if this requires help from a member of staff. Venous stasis should be kept to a minimum using elastic stockings or a one way stretch bandage (Chapter 10). Some clinicians recommend that patients at high risk from venous thrombosis should be treated with heparin given subcutaneously in a dose of 5,000 iu twice daily. The problems of multiple pathology in old people are such that prophylactic anti-coagulants can have no more than a very limited role to play in this situation. Once the thrombosis has occurred patients should be treated with a combination of heparin followed by a coumarin anticoagulant. Where there has been a pulmonary embolism, anticoagulants should again be used. Other supportive measures including relief of pain, administration of oxygen or even thoracic surgery may be indicated.

## Further reading

Block E R (1979) Pitfalls in diagnosing and managing pulmonary disease. *Geriatrics*, **34**, 70–80

Campbell E J & Lefrak S S (1978) How ageing affects the structure and function of the respiratory system. *Geriatrics*, **33**, 68–74

Iseman M D (1980) Tuberculosis in the elderly: treating the "white plague". *Geriatrics*, **35**, 90–107

Riordan J F (1979) Carcinoma of the bronchus. *Br J Hosp Med*, **22**, 120–127

Webster J & Davison R (1977) Aspiration pneumonitis: a serious problem. *Geriatrics*, **32**, 42–47

# CHAPTER 12

# The Gastrointestinal Tract and Anaemia

## Alimentary disease

**Mouth and teeth.** Some of the problems relating to nutrition have already been mentioned in Chapter 6 but the state of the mouth and teeth may also have an important influence in this area. Dental care of the elderly is often neglected. Nevertheless, carious and broken teeth or ill-fitting dentures are uncomfortable and may give rise to oral ulceration. As the majority of the elderly are edentulous, most of the treatment relates to the stomatognathic changes which occur; consequently, denture cleaning, relining, rebasing, easing and repairing should be considered in all those who wear false teeth. It should be remembered that some elderly people are sensitive to modern plastics used in the manufacture of false teeth, so that repairing and refitting old dentures may be better than making new sets.

Many old people complain of a sore tongue or oral ulcers. While these may be related to dental trauma (see above) other causes such as vitamin deficiency (Chapter 6), anaemia (this chapter) and other blood diseases, as well as aphthous ulceration and infection, may occur. Treatment should be directed to the cause.

Aphthous ulceration may respond to hydrocortisone pellets (Corlan) or local insufflation of disodium chromoglycate (Intal) which can be most effective in relieving pain and discomfort.

A sore tongue may sometimes be associated with drug therapy, neurosis, depressive illness and mouth infection. Perhaps the commonest infection is monilia (*Candida albicans*), commonly known as thrush. It should always be suspected if white patches are seen on the tongue, throat or buccal cavity. Diagnosis is confirmed by culture of mouth or throat swabs, and treatment with local applications of nystatin given in the form of paints and lozenges. The condition is common in those with severe debility, illness or bacterial infection.

**Hiatus hernia, chest pain and dysphagia** (Case 6). Well over half of all elderly people have a hiatus hernia or free oesophageal regurgitation. This can cause trouble in a variety of ways.

(a) *Chest pain.* It is often difficult to distinguish the chest pain of hiatus hernia from that of coronary artery disease. Both conditions are so common in old age that they often occur in the same individual, and the doctor should always keep this in mind before embarking on treatment for one or other of these disorders.

The pain of hiatus hernia can be relieved using a variety of antacids. If it is severe and persistent the $H_2$ receptor antagonists cimetidine and ranitidine are extremely effective. However, before these are used the diagnosis should be confirmed by radiology or endoscopy. It is even more important that the patient should adopt the correct posture. Elevation of the oesophagus above the level of the stomach prevents the reflux of acid into the former. At night, this is achieved by elevating the head of the bed on blocks. Propping the patient up with pillows increases intra-abdominal pressure, which is sufficient to force acid into the oesophagus against gravity. Surgery should be considered if medical and conservative measures fail to relieve symptoms and if anaemia does not respond to iron.

(b) *Difficulty in swallowing (dysphagia).* Damage to the wall of the oesophagus by acid may cause narrowing with dysphagia (fibrous stricture); this symptom often indicates other serious diseases and should never be neglected. It can be treated initially by mechanical dilatation, but with repeated dilatation the risk of rupture increases. Cancer of the oesophagus itself, pressure from enlarged mediastinal glands or tumours of the lung also cause the symptoms. The prospect of a slow death from pain and starvation in this situation is so appalling that the advice of a surgeon should always be sought, no matter how old and frail the patient.

External pressure may also be caused by a dilated arteriosclerotic blood vessel such as the aorta or the inominate artery. When this happens no treatment apart from reassurance is necessary.

A barium swallow in a very old patient may coincidentally show abnormal oesophageal contractions. Peristaltic activity is lost and replaced by inco-ordinated contractions giving the appearance of a 'corkscrew' oesophagus. The appearance is of little clinical relevance and is best ignored.

**Peptic ulcer** (Cases 3, 6). Duodenal and gastric ulcers reach a peak incidence in middle age but remain sufficiently common in old age to cause a lot of trouble. They may present in a variety of ways, particularly with general malaise, vomiting, epigastric pain and haemorrhage.

(a) *Pain*. This symptom is often absent because the elderly may have an increased threshold to painful stimuli and a reduced inflammatory response to tissue injury. Peptic ulceration may thus remain an unsuspected cause of weight loss, anaemia or even confusion in many old people.

(b) *Haemorrhage*. This is the most serious complication of peptic ulceration in old age, and when acute is associated with an extremely high mortality which is probably due to the high incidence of co-existent disease rather than to ageing itself. The only way of minimising the risk is by subjecting the patient to immediate surgery. Bleeding is unlikely to stop spontaneously and any delay will merely make the patient even less fit for an operation. If, for any reason, a decision is taken not to operate, the patient should not be put on to a massive and prolonged blood transfusion as this will merely prolong dying rather than save life.

Chronic haemorrhage giving rise to iron deficiency anaemia is also common (see below: hypochromic anaemia), and may sometimes be associated with a giant gastric ulcer; this can be difficult to differentiate from gastric cancer.

*Investigation and treatment.*   Diagnosis, particularly in the case of the giant gastric ulcer, can only be made with certainty by gastroscopy and biopsy of the ulcer with a fibreoptic gastroscope. If adequately premedicated with diazepam, the elderly often sleep throughout the procedure and remember nothing afterwards apart from the unpleasantness of the local anaesthetic throat spray. Other investigatory procedures, particularly radiology, may also be helpful. Investigation of gastric secretions is of less value because about 30 per cent of the elderly have achlorhydria and 40 per cent of these have chronic atrophic gastritis.

While antacids still have a part to play in the management of peptic ulcers; the most effective treatment is to use an $H_2$ receptor antagonist. Cimetidine is less expensive than ranitidine, but has the disadvantage of occasionally causing confusion, and interacting with other drugs. In practice these problems rarely arise, even in old age so that cimetidine remains the drug of first choice. Surgery is only indicated when acute haemorrhage or pyloric stenosis occurs.

**Gastric cancer** (Case 3).   The symptoms of this condition also are often vague and ill-defined, varying from a 'failure to thrive' to frank depression or even an acute confusional state. The standard explanation is that these symptoms are produced by toxins released by tumour cells.

Surgery has little effect on the life expectancy of patients with gastric carcinoma. It should only be used in the elderly to prevent or relieve intolerable symptoms such as those due to pyloric obstruction; relief of mental or physical impairment may be yet another reason. The management of terminal illness is considered in Chapter 15.

*Previous gastric surgery.* Any list of elderly patients 'at risk' in the community should include people who have had surgery for peptic ulceration. Alteration of the anatomy or function of the upper alimentary tract can cause malabsorption of a wide range of nutrients, which in the elderly can produce the effects of severe weight loss, severe anaemia, and loss of bone mass with an increased attendant risk of fractures. Less specifically, the already decreased resistance to infection is accentuated so that the reactivation of a long quiescent focus of pulmonary tuberculosis may occur.

Complications often develop 20 or 30 years after an operation when the episode has been forgotten by doctor and patient alike. Failure to identify the problem condemns the patient to chronic ill health and may result in permanent disability.

**Malabsorption** (Case 7). Malabsorption may occur in old people, as in any other age group. Common causes of this include gluten-sensitive enteropathy, diverticula, disease of the duodenum or jejunum, and previous gastric surgery. Complex investigation may be necessary to elucidate the problem. The condition is often missed, associated weight loss being attributed to a poor diet, but as dietary deficiency is rare in active old people any weight loss requires urgent medical investigation. Treatment should be directed to the cause and complications (Chapter 7: metabolic bone disease).

**Gallbladder disease** (Case 6). Gallbladder disease is common in the elderly, occurring in 25 per cent of men and women over the age of 70. It is often asymptomatic, producing no more than an occasional episode of flatulence after a particularly heavy meal. If, however, the condition does flare up as gallbladder obstruction and inflammation it can be particularly unpleasant. It may also present atypically as an acute illness with few abdominal symptoms. Mortality bears a direct relationship to the age and disability of the patient.

Surgery should only be undertaken if gallstones are causing symptoms. A large proportion of old people have gallstones which are asymptomatic. Preventive surgery on all of them would produce a higher morbidity and mortality than leaving them untreated until symptoms arise.

If the gallstones consist of cholesterol, and the gall-bladder is still functioning, it often is possible to dissolve the stones with oral doses of chenodeoxycholic acid. However, the process takes a long time and treatment has to be continued indefinitely, so that most clinicians only use it if the patient is too frail for surgery.

If the gallstone is in the common bile duct it is sometimes possible to extract it using an endoscope. Again, this is a useful procedure in the elderly patient too frail for conventional surgery.

**Jaundice** (Case 6). Table 12.1 lists the relative incidences for the major causes of jaundice in the elderly hospital patients: the particular importance of drugs as a cause of jaundice should be noted. Many potentially hepatotoxic drugs are in wide general use in geriatric practice, including the anti-convulsant phenytoin, phenothiazine tranquillisers, the anabolic derivatives of testosterone and the oral hypoglycaemic, chlorpropamide. The efficacy of these agents overrides their hepatotoxicity. A careful drug history, however, should be elicited in every case of jaundice. This can usefully be supplemented by a careful search round the house, for old people are notorious hoarders and may be taking tablets prescribed many years previously either for themselves or for some long dead relative.

**Appendicitis.** As with other causes of abdominal pain, the symptoms of appendicitis in the elderly are often mild and poorly localised (Chapter 2). The vague abdominal ache may be attributed to constipation and either ignored or treated with laxatives. Poor tissue resistance results in a rapid evolution from local sepsis to generalised peritonitis so that by the time a doctor is consulted the patient may be moribund. If a prohibitively high mortality is to be avoided it is essential that the condition should be over- rather than under-diagnosed. An unnecessary medical visit or, indeed, an unnecessary operation is far preferable to a delay in diagnosis where the condition is present.

**Diverticulosis coli.** Almost half the population over 70 years of age have diverticular disease of the colon. The symptoms are usually minimal but

Table 12.1  Causes of Jaundice in the Elderly (Eastwood 1971)

| Condition | Percentage |
|---|---|
| Cancer of biliary tract | 22 |
| Calculi in biliary tract | 16 |
| Cirrhosis | 10 |
| Hepatic secondaries | 12 |
| Hepatitis | 15 |
| Hepatic abscess | 0 |
| Haemolysis | 5 |
| Drugs | 21 |

complications such as massive haemorrhage, or abscess formation, are fairly common.

The disease is probably a consequence of the highly refined low-roughage diets taken in Western society. Muscle contraction in the colonic wall is normally used to push faeces along the lumen. When faeces are low in bulk, muscle contraction merely increases the intraluminal pressure which, ultimately, results in the herniation of gut mucosa through areas of weakness in the muscle coat with diverticulum formation.

The condition can be prevented or minimised by increasing the amount of roughage in the diet. Bran is a useful source of roughage; tastes vary, but most patients prefer to take it mixed with ordinary meals, and a dose of one tablespoonful up to three times daily is usual.

**Cancer of colon and rectum.**   Cancer of the lower alimentary tract some-times present dramatically as an acute obstruction; more often, it results in a gradual deterioration in health associated with a change in bowel habit. As with cancer of the stomach, changes in mood and cognitive function are common. These symptoms are all too commonly attributed to the inevitable consequences of ageing and are either not treated at all, or attacked with a rigorous regime of laxatives and enemas. A sudden change in bowel function may be due to faecal impaction, but the possi-bility of cancer should always be considered and, if necessary, excluded by endoscopic and radiological investigation.

**Ulcerative colitis, Crohn's disease, ischaemic colitis.**   Each of these con-ditions may occur in old age and ischaemic colitis is particularly associ-ated with the ageing process. Diagnosis of the first two conditions must be made by biopsy of the abnormal bowel – the radiological appearance of the barium enema shows a loss of the haustral pattern while the colon has a 'thumb-printing' appearance in ischaemic colitis.

**Rectal prolapse.**   A common and very uncomfortable and distressing condition. It is frequently found in women and may relate to damage to the anal sphincter which can occur in child bearing; it results in faecal incontinence or soiling. Treatment is aimed at either restoring anal sphincter tone or reducing the size of the anus by inserting a silver wire. Thereafter, stools must be kept soft and constipation avoided (*see* Chap-ter 14).

**Constipation.**   This is considered in detail in Chapter 14.

## Anaemia (Case 3)

The incidence of anaemia depends upon the sample studied, as well as on the haemoglobin level below which anaemia is said to occur. The level of

12 g/dl is probably the best single level for the definition of anaemia in old age. Community surveys show an incidence of between 5 and 15 per cent, while the incidence in elderly subjects admitted to hospital is considerably greater, being 25 per cent in men and 40 per cent in women.

*Investigation.* Investigation should start with a detailed history. Particular points requiring consideration include alimentary symptoms, dietary habits, previous gastro-intestinal surgery and analgesic or steroid intake. A detailed physical examination, including rectal examination is, of course, essential, and where necessary this should be followed by laboratory investigations (Chapter 3). Figure 12.1 details a rational approach to this problem. Investigation should also be governed by whether action will be taken if a test is positive: a surgeon is unlikely to resect a carcinoma of caecum in a grossly demented, bedfast and doubly incontinent 95-year-old man.

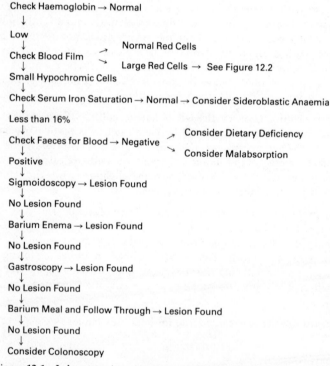

Figure 12.1   Laboratory investigation of anaemia. (*Note:* The flow chart assumes that the clinical features were negative. Where these are positive, many of the steps may be by-passed.)

**Hypochromic anaemia.** Iron deficiency is by far the most common cause of anaemia in old age; it is occasionally due to dietary deficiency but is much more often a result of gastro-intestinal blood loss. The wide range of alimentary lesions responsible for this blood loss have been described earlier in this chapter. Many pain-relieving tablets may also cause bleeding, the most widely used of which are aspirin and its related compounds. Agents such as phenylbutazone or indomethacin and other non-steroidal anti-inflammatory drugs are equally dangerous. A considerable amount of persuasion is necessary to induce patients to stop taking these drugs to which they are often habituated. They find considerable difficulty in converting to a safer agent such as paracetamol. Paracetamol is often combined with other substances eg. dextropropoxyphene (Distalgesic). These may also cause habituation and contribute to confusional states when combined with other drugs which act on the central nervous system. Steroids also cause bleeding by increasing acid secretion and inducing peptic ulceration, and this is one of the many reasons for avoiding or minimising the use of these agents in the elderly.

**Macrocytic anaemia.** If the blood film contains large red cells (macrocytes) the bone marrow should be aspirated (Fig. 12.2), and if microscopic examination shows large red cell precursors (megaloblasts), a diagnosis of vitamin $B_{12}$ or folic acid deficiency is then likely. This can be checked by measuring the blood levels of these two vitamins. $B_{12}$ deficiency may be due to a failure of intrinsic factor production by the gastric mucosa, or the over-growth of $B_{12}$ metabolising bacteria in duodenal or jejunal diverticula. The tests used in differentiating the two forms of $B_{12}$ deficiency are outlined in Figure 12.2 (details of the test will be found in most modern textbooks of gastroenterology). $B_{12}$ deficiency is treated by injections of cyanocobalamin: a simple regime is to give $1,000\,\mu g$ on three consecutive days and then $250\,\mu g$ at three-weekly intervals.

Folic acid deficiency in old age is usually related to defective nutrition. It is rarely an isolated finding, in that it usually is accompanied by chronic ill health, severe disability or mental impairment. All are situations in which folate intake is likely to be deficient. The red cell folate concentration should be estimated to confirm the diagnosis.

Treatment is by folic acid in a dose of 20 mg daily. Serum $B_{12}$ levels should always be measured before folic acid supplements are started because old people are particularly susceptible to the mental and neurological effects of $B_{12}$ depletion, which will be accentuated if folic acid is used injudiciously.

**Normochromic normocytic anaemia.** Many old people suffer from a mild anaemia in which the red cells are normal in size (normocytic) and contain normal quantities of haemoglobin (normochromic). It is often due

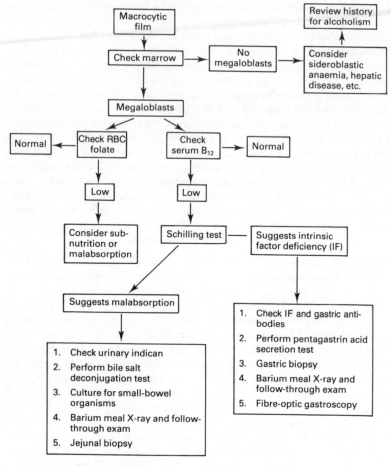

Figure 12.2   Investigation of macrocytic anaemia

to a wide range of chronic conditions, including rheumatoid arthritis, tuberculosis, renal failure, multiple myeloma and carcinomatosis. Identification of this type of anaemia should lead to a painstaking search for one or more of these disorders (Fig. 12.3). Treatment of the anaemia usually involves treatment of the primary condition.

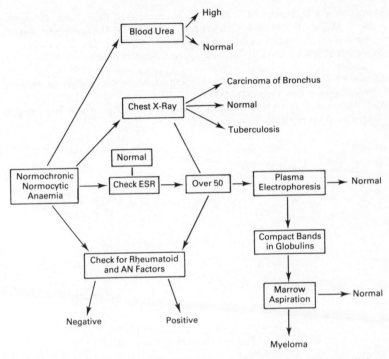

Figure 12.3  Investigation of normochromic normocytic anaemia. (*Note:* If all these investigations are negative, look for evidence of carcinomatosis. Common primary sources are the breast, kidney, prostate and thyroid. Alimentary carcinoma more usually causes hypochromic anaemia, but there are exceptions.)

## Further reading

Exton-Smith A N & Caird F I (1980) *Metabolic and Nutritional Disorders in the Elderly*. Bristol: Wright

Fish S F (1975) . . . in a good age. *Brit Dent J*, **138**, 473–479

Hollis J & Castell D O (1974) Oesophageal function in elderly men: a new look at presbyesophagus. *Ann Intern Med*, **80**, 371–374

Hellemans, J, Vantrappen & Pelemans W (1982) Oesophageal disorders in old people. In *Recent Advances in Geriatric Medicine 2*. Isaacs B (ed) Edinburgh: Churchill Livingstone

James O F W (1983) Gastrointestinal and liver function in old age. *Clin. Gastroenterol*, **12**, 671–691

MacLennan W J, Andrews G R, MacLeod C C & Caird F I (1973) Anaemia in the elderly. *Quart J Med*, **42**, 1–13

Montgomery R D, Haeney M R, Ross I N, Sammons H G, Barford A V, Balakrishnan S, Mayer P P, Culank L S, Field J & Gesling P (1978) The ageing gut: a study of intestinal absorption in relation to the elderly. *Quart J Med*, **47**, 197–211

Nettle P & Hughes E (1981) Gallstones: operate, dissolve or leave alone? *Drugs*, **21**, 302–308

Richter J F & Castell D O (1981) Current approaches in the medical treatment of oesophageal reflux. *Drugs*, **21**, 283–291

Van Bezooijen C F A (1983) Pharmacological, Morphological and Physiological Aspects of Liver Aging. Rijswijk: Eurage

# CHAPTER 13

# Homeostasis

### Thyrotoxicosis (hyperthyroidism)

Thyroid disease is common in old age but is often mis-diagnosed. The classical features of the disorder include an increased appetite, excessive sweating, preference for cold weather, and loose bowel motions, but these are often minimal or absent in old people. Although the general features of thyrotoxicosis are diminished, cardiovascular abnormalities are accentuated; these include tachycardia, atrial fibrillation and heart failure. Occasionally the patient may be lethargic and withdrawn (apathetic thyrotoxicosis) so that the doctor has the embarrassment of sending a specimen of blood off to the laboratory with the query of hypothyroidism only to find that the results suggest thyrotoxicosis. Details of the appropriate laboratory tests are described in Chapter 3.

**Treatment.** Old people are normally treated either with anti-thyroid drugs such as carbimazole or with radioactive iodine, thyroidectomy rarely being necessary. Carbimazole produces a reduction of thyroid function over the course of several weeks. If this happens remission is usually maintained when the drug is withdrawn twelve to eighteen months later, but unfortunately some old people do not respond to treatment.

Radioactive iodine therapy is rapidly and universally effective in old age. Eventually, however, the majority of cases develop myxoedema (hypothyroidism). This is no disadvantage if follow-up is adequate, but old people often forget or are unable to keep appointments, so that they frequently become hypothyroid. This can only be avoided if patients are placed on an 'at risk' register and supervised by district nurses and health visitors (Chapter 1).

### Myxoedema (hypothyroidism)

The diagnosis of hypothyroidism is equally difficult because it mimics many of the features naturally associated with ageing (Table 13.1). Although this means that thyroid function tests are over-requested and are often negative, the cost of the tests is more than balanced by the disastrous consequences of missing the diagnosis. Details of the laboratory investigation for hypothyroidism are given in Chapter 3.

Table 13.1   Clinical Features in Ageing and Hypothyroidism

| Clinical feature | Ageing | Hypothyroidism |
|---|---|---|
| Coarse skin | Present | Present |
| Hair loss | Present | Present |
| Mental slowness | Often present | Present |
| Hoarseness | Sometimes present | Present |
| Reduction in sweating | Present | Present |
| Intolerance of cold | Present | Present |
| Poor peripheral circulation | Present | Present |
| Reduced heart rate | Often present | Present |
| Unsteadiness | Present (usually non-specific) | Present (usually) |
| Constipation | Often present | Present |
| Poor appetite | Often present | Present |

**Treatment.**   Hypothyroidism is treated by the administration of thyroxine. The susceptibility of the myocardium to the hormone is increased, probably due to a combination of coronary artery disease, cardiac amyloidosis and potassium depletion. Extreme caution must be used when giving thyroxine; the initial dose should be 50 μg daily, increasing by 50 μg daily after four to six weeks. Ideally, the patient should be kept in hospital and have regular electrocardiographs for the first two or three weeks of treatment, but social and clinical pressures on beds make this difficult. Caution over the cardiovascular effects of thyroxine must be balanced against the serious consequences of replacement therapy being inadequate. This can be avoided by re-checking thyroxine levels once dosage has been stabilised. Usually this lies between 100 μg and 150 μg daily.

The two main complications of hypothyroidism in old age are mental impairment and hypothermia. The response of mental impairment to thyroxine is often disappointing, but a gratifying improvement is occasionally encountered. A possible explanation for the permanent effect of hypothyroidism on cerebral function in the elderly is that ageing is associated with a decline in the reserve capacity of the brain. Destruction of minimal numbers of brain cells, in this situation, may be sufficient to make the difference between competence in everyday activities and moderately severe dementia. Myxoedematous hypothermia is best considered in the general context of hypothermia.

## Hypothermia

Hypothermia is defined as being present when the temperature of the central body falls below 35°C. Exposure to cold is the most important causative factor. Social factors such as inadequate heating, poor housing insulation or inappropriate clothing are important, but they only produce hypothermia where they are coupled with damage to endogenous temperature regulation. The wide range of factors responsible for this are listed in Table 13.2.

The clinical signs are vague: mild hypothermia may produce pallor, apathy and tachyardia; little else seems amiss. The patient rarely complains of feeling cold. Below 32°C physical deterioration is more obvious, the signs including a slow irregular pulse, a slow respiratory rate, muscle rigidity, peripheral or facial oedema, and hypotension; the level of consciousness varies between drowsiness and deep coma.

The essentials for diagnosis include a high index of suspicion and a low-reading thermometer. The axillary temperature should be checked and where this is less than 35°C the rectal temperature should be taken; this differentiates between a low skin temperature due to peripheral vasoconstriction and a breakdown in the thermoregulation of the central body core.

Patients with mild hypothermia, if identified and treated, make an uneventful recovery. Mortality is high when the body temperature is less than 32°C, the death rate exceeding 50 per cent. Complications are related

Table 13.2  Endogenous Causes of Hypothermia

*Brain damage*
  Cerebrovascular disease
  Senile dementia
  Parkinsonism

*Suppression of temperature control*
  Phenothiazine tranquillisers
  Barbiturates
  Tricyclic antidepressants
  Anticholinergic smooth-muscle
    relaxants
  Alcohol

*Immobility*
  Neurological disease
  Osteoarthritis
  Rheumatoid arthritis

*Acute illness*
  Coronary thrombosis
  Pneumonia
  Pulmonary embolism
  Fractured hip
  Gastrointestinal haemorrhage
  Cerebrovascular accident

*Endocrine disease*
  Hypothyroidism
  Adrenal failure
  Diabetes mellitus

*Increased temperature loss*
  Diminished insulation due to
    loss of body fat
  Skin disease associated with
    hyperaemia
  Large leg ulcers

to a disturbance of cardiac function, increased intravascular coagulation and an impaired immunological response to infection (Table 13.3). Systemic and focal manifestations are often silent with minimal symptoms since the body is unable to respond to these pathological conditions.

Table 13.3   Complications of Hypothermia

| | |
|---|---|
| *Vascular* | *Alimentary* |
| Mesenteric thrombosis | Pancreatitis |
| Peripheral gangrene | |
| Coronary thrombosis | *Renal* |
| | Acute renal failure |
| *Respiratory* | |
| Pneumonia | |

Treatment with hot water bottles or an electric blanket is a highly effective way of killing patients with hypothermia because it induces peripheral vasodilatation and the heart is then incapable of maintaining an adequate output for the expanded circulatory system. Hypotension, shock and death are the inevitable consequences.

Reheating must take place very gradually. In the mild case this can be done by placing the patient in a warm room, and giving him hot drinks. Spirits should never be used because they produce peripheral vasodilation which causes further heat loss and a further reduction in core temperature. Thermal blankets may cause shock by too rapid re-warming and should not be used on old people. In severe cases, with temperatures below 32°C, admission to hospital and intensive care is essential. Even here, however, treatment should be conservative. There is no evidence that techniques such as heating with a body cradle, mediastinal irrigation, or extracorporeal perfusion produce a lower mortality than gradual re-warming.

Reheating should be combined with several ancillary measures: antibiotics are given to prevent or control the otherwise inevitable chest infection, and dehydration is corrected with appropriate intravenous fluids. Intubation should be avoided since it may provoke ventricular fibrillation and a defibrillator should be available.

Death from hypothermia is best minimised by preventing the condition and old people at risk must be visited regularly, as well as being given advice on clothing, heating and insulation. Disabled people should receive adequate domestic support either from home helps or neighbours. People with low incomes should be advised on their rights to supplementary heating allowances and supplementary benefits.

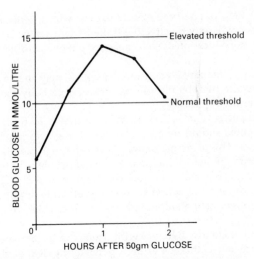

Figure 13.1    Effect of renal threshold of glycosuria
in a patient with impaired glucose tolerance

## Diabetes (Case 1)

**Screening and prevalence.**   Ageing is associated with a decrease in the control of carbohydrate metabolism, which may be the result of changes in the organs which control metabolic processes, other than the islets of Langerhans. Further, there may be an increased tissue resistance to insulin rather than a major change in insulin release from the pancreas, or even the production of an insulin antagonist.

Checking urine for glucose is of limited value as a screening test of diabetes in old people because many old people have impaired renal function. In particular, the filtration of urine through the glomeruli is reduced and this has the effect of increasing the renal threshold for glucose, namely, the blood level of glucose at which glucose first appears in the urine. In this situation a patient with impaired glucose tolerance may not have glycosuria (Fig. 13.1). Diabetes can only be excluded in old people by investigating blood glucose levels (Chapter 3). The results of glucose tolerance tests should be viewed with caution unless the patient has been on a 300 g carbohydrate diet for three days before the test is done: this is a lot of carbohydrate for an old person.

## Treatment

(a) *Diet.* Glucose intolerance is often relatively mild in the elderly and may be controlled by diet alone. 1,000 calories and 100 g of carbohydrate may be sufficient in an obese elderly patient with recent-onset diabetes. This approach will only be effective if the patient can be persuaded of its importance; the education of well-meaning but over-indulgent relatives is also essential.

(b) *Exercise.* Graduated, monitored exercise may increase tissue sensitivity to insulin thereby improving control of carbohydrate metabolism and lowering insulin levels.

(c) *Oral hypoglycaemics* (Case 1). When a diet is ineffective oral hypoglycaemic agents should be added, of which the sulphonylureas are the most effective. The principal danger is that hypoglycaemia may occur if the dose is too high, which happens when old people excrete drugs poorly so that toxic levels result. The risk can be minimised by giving a drug with a short duration of action such as tolbutamide or glipizide, and for this reason longer-acting sulphonylureas such as chlorpropamide should be avoided if possible.

The control of elderly diabetics with drugs can be extremely difficult. If a patient is treated so that his urine is persistently clear of glucose he may run the risk of hypoglycaemic attacks. The alternative is to allow him to have a trace of glucose in his urine. If he has a high renal threshold for glucose this may represent poor control of his diabetes and the risk from complications will increase. There is no easy answer to the problem. A reasonable compromise can often be reached by performing serial blood glucose level tests in hospital and relating these to drug dosage and urine testing. Where this is done the patient and his relatives should be warned that any change in diet may upset the balance, and necessitate further medical assessment.

The biguanide hypoglycaemics have the advantage, over the sulphonylureas, of not producing hypoglycaemia. However, many old people have impaired renal function and there is a substantial risk that the biguanides in general and phenformin in particular may cause a serious disturbance of acid/base balance in such susceptible individuals. They are best avoided, therefore, in the elderly.

(d) *Insulin.* Some elderly diabetic patients require insulin, the preparations used being those for any age group. Administration causes certain problems in old age, for the elderly are particularly sensitive to sudden changes in blood glucose levels, which may provoke intermittent bouts of confusion. Stabilisation is best achieved by serial blood glucose estimations, taken at four-hourly intervals between 8 am and 12 midnight. Unexpected blood glucose peaks and troughs are often demonstrated by this method.

Disability complicates insulin therapy. Patients with arthritic hands or impaired vision often find it impossible to inject themselves with the right dose of insulin, and people with mental impairment have the same problem. This can result in a vicious circle of confusion due to inadequate control with consequent wrong dosage, resulting in even worse control with even more confusion.

The only solution here is to place the control of insulin into the hands of a responsible person, who could be a relative, friend or neighbour, or the district nurse. In some situations effective supervision may only be achieved by admission to warden-supported or residential accommodation.

**Complications of diabetes** (Case 1).   The complications of diabetes make an important contribution to the wide range of disabilities found in the elderly, the more common of which are listed in Table 13.4. There is now good evidence that the onset and progress of many such conditions can be prevented or slowed by careful control of the blood glucose concentration.

The investigation and management of the ocular, respiratory, renal, cardiac and cerebral manifestations of diabetes is that for any age group. Involvement of the feet presents particular problems, for the patient is often afflicted by the combination of neuropathy and poor peripheral circulation. Identification of the nerve disease is difficult because many relatively healthy old people exhibit an impaired sense of vibration and no ankle tendon reflexes. Again, a large proportion of old people have absent peripheral pulses.

Probably the best approach is to observe extreme caution in caring for the feet of all elderly diabetics. All local treatment should be undertaken by a trained chiropodist, footwear should be comfortable and well-fitting, and local infections or ulcers should receive prompt attention, for if these

Table 13.4   Complications of Diabetes

| | |
|---|---|
| *Vascular* | *Ophthalmic* |
| Cerebrovascular disease | Cataracts |
| Coronary artery disease | Retinal damage |
| Peripheral vascular disease | |
| Postural hypotension | *Neurological* |
| | Peripheral neuropathy |
| *Infections* | Flaccid urinary bladder |
| Pulmonary tuberculosis | Defective autonomic nervous system |
| Pneumonia | |
| Urinary infections | *Renal* |
| Thrush (mouth, vagina or skin) | Protein leakage |
| Gangrene | Chronic renal infection |
| | Renal nephropathy |
| *Alimentary* | |
| Malabsorption | |
| Diarrhoea | |

are neglected, they may quickly spread to produce extensive necrosis and gangrene. A superficial lesion should be treated with a dry dressing; if it is deeper and if there is pus and necrotic tissue, gauze soaked in cetrimide should be used. Systemic antibiotics are helpful in preventing the spread of the condition.

There is increasing recognition that diabetes often compromises bladder innervation in the elderly. The bladder becomes large and atonic and a persistent, dribbling incontinence is the usual result. The diagnosis is easily identified by performing cystometrography in suspected cases. Bladder tonus may be increased using bethanechol (*cf*. Chapter 14).

**Diabetic coma.** As in other groups, old people may present in diabetic coma or pre-coma, with a blood glucose level that is grossly elevated and a serious disturbance of acid-base balance. The management of this condition is that for any age group. Sometimes, however, the blood-sugar can reach very high levels without any dramatic symptoms and without a significant change in acid-base balance.

The principal signs of the condition are a gradual deterioration in consciousness and dehydration. Hyperglycaemia has a very variable effect on mental function and some people only start to become drowsy with blood sugars in excess of 50 mmol/l. Dehydration, again, is easily mistaken for the lax and inelastic skin often found in old age. It is not surprising then, that a hyperglycaemic crisis often goes unnoticed by relatives, and even district nurses and health visitors, until it has reached a very advanced stage. It is for these reasons, perhaps, that the condition carries a 50 per cent mortality. The condition is known as hyperosmolar non-ketotic diabetic coma.

Hyperglycaemic coma is treated with the rapid infusion of fluid either as saline or glucose in a weak saline solution. A relatively small dose of insulin is often all that is necessary. If the patient survives, the result may be extremely gratifying in that she is restored from being a rambling and bedfast vegetable to an alert and useful member of society.

## Renal function

Increasing age is associated with a considerable alteration in renal function. Cross-sectional studies have shown a progressive decline in both the filtration of urine through the glomeruli and the excretion and reabsorption of substances by the renal tubules. This is partly due to an age-related cell death causing a decline in the numbers of functioning glomeruli and tubules. The process is often accelerated by the wide range of diseases which occur in old age, including high blood pressure, chronic renal infections, diabetes and urinary obstruction.

The age-related decline in renal function has important clinical implications in the management of illness in the elderly. The first of these is that
the kidneys have virtually no functional reserve. Any fall in the flow of
blood and plasma through the kidneys is likely to result in a rapidly rising
blood urea; common causes of this include blood loss, coronary thrombosis and dehydration, and the last may be the result of vomiting, diarrhoea, diabetic coma or the injudicious use of diuretics. For these reasons,
seemingly trivial illnesses should never be ignored in the elderly, for a
mild gastro-intestinal upset can rapidly progress to coma and irreversible
renal shutdown.

Many drugs are excreted by the kidney. The reduction in renal function
in the elderly often causes a build-up of drug blood levels. Drugs affected
in this way include digoxin, chlorpropamide and phenobarbitone. Some
drugs which are safe in young healthy individuals may have a toxic effect
on the kidneys where there is pre-existing renal impairment. Important
examples include the first generation cephalosporins and the tetra-
cyclines.

Renal impairment is only part of the explanation for old people rapidly
developing fluid and electrolyte imbalance. Another problem is that of
impaired thirst sensation. The exact mechanism behind this is obscure,
but there is no doubt that some old people abstain from water for long
periods without experiencing thirst, and the condition is particularly
prominent in patients with organic brain disease. The effect of dehydration may be further accentuated by impaired anti-diuretic hormone
(ADH) secretion. There is good evidence for an age-related decline in
ADH release from the posterior pituitary which may, in part, explain the
inability of the elderly kidney to concentrate urine.

The message to emerge from these phenomena is that fluid balance
should play a very important part in the management of all elderly
patients. The clinical signs of dehydration are difficult to detect in old age;
they may be mimicked by the inelastic skin and by the loss of intraorbital
tissue so often found in the elderly. Reliance must be placed on measuring
blood urea concentrations and initiating fluid balance charts. Fluid charts
should be used on all patients with an important elevation in their blood
urea. These can be difficult to record if the patient is incontinent and
serious consideration should always be given to catheterisation, but here
the dangers of urinary tract infection must be weighed against those of
being unable to measure fluid balance.

### Urinary tract infection

A large proportion of elderly patients admitted to a geriatric ward have
infected urine, and the decision has to be made whether or not every case

should be treated. In the first place, an accurate diagnosis must be made, but this is dependent upon collecting an uncontaminated specimen of urine from the bladder. Collection of a mid-stream specimen of urine usually meets this requirement in men, but the technique is much more difficult in elderly women. Over 50 per cent of specimens collected in this way are likely to be contaminated unless perineal and vulval cleansing have been very thorough.

One way of avoiding contamination is to aspirate urine through a neadle inserted into the bladder above the pubic symphysis. If the bladder is sufficiently distended to allow easy penetration the procedure is not particularly unpleasant and is free from serious side effects. Many old ladies empty their bladder too frequently for this precondition so that the technique is only successful in about 50 per cent of cases.

An alternative approach is to make use of Alexa microcatheters. Here, a small catheter connected to a collection bag is inserted into the urethra and as soon as the bag is filled with urine the catheter is withdrawn. Experience has shown that this procedure rarely introduces infection into the bladder and that it gives a degree of diagnostic accuracy similar to suprapubic aspiration.

Urinary tract infection, once identified, should only be treated if it is giving rise to symptoms. Asymptomatic bacteriuria in the elderly is not often associated with renal infection and is rarely responsible for incontinence, although it may often be associated with it (Chapter 14). Antibiotic therapy will inevitably produce organisms highly resistant to all but the most toxic agents, and treatment should be reserved for patients with systemic or local symptoms. Ampicillin, co-trimoxazole and nalidixic acid are all suitable agents. Tetracycline and first generation cephalosporins (other than cephedrine) are nephrotoxic in patients with poor renal function in the elderly and should not be used. Nitrofurantion should also be avoided, because its neurological side effects are particularly common in old age. Once started, treatment should be continued for at least seven days.

## Further reading

Bahemuka M & Hodkinson H M (1975) Screening for hypothyroidism in elderly patients. Br Med J, 2, 601–603

Britton K E, Ellis S M, Miralles J M, Quinn V, Cayley A C D, Brown B L & Ekins R P (1975) Is 'T$_4$ toxicosis' a normal biochemical finding in elderly women? Lancet, ii, 141–142

Burrows A W, Shakespear R A, Hesch R D, Cooper E, Aickin C M & Burke C W (1975) Thyroid hormones in the elderly sick: 'T$_4$ euthyroidism'. Br Med J, 4, 437–439

Butterfield W J H, Keen H & Whicklow M J (1967) Renal glucose threshold variations with age. *Br Med J*, **4**, 505–507

Collins K J, Dore C, Exton-Smith A N, Fox R H, MacDonald I C & Woodward P M (1977) Accidental hypothermia and impaired temperature homeostasis in the elderly. *Br Med J*, **1**, 353–356

Hodkinson H M & Irvine R E (1985) Thyroid disease in old age. In Brocklehurst J C (ed) *Textbook of Geriatric Medicine & Gerontology*. Edinburgh: Churchill Livingstone

MacCurdy D K (1970) Hyperosmolar hyperglycaemic nonketotic coma. *Med Clin N Amer*, **54**, 683–699

# CHAPTER 14

# Incontinence

In Chapter 2 we briefly considered the problem of social acceptability. Incontinence, whether urinary or faecal, is a common cause of social rejection as well as distress to the patient and those close to him. It is often considered a natural concomitant of ageing. This is wrong: it should be considered a remediable condition in all patients who suffer from it, even though we fail to cure some.

## Urinary incontinence

Incontinence of urine is a problem which affects approximately 40 per cent of patients admitted to a geriatric ward. It is often due to the restriction to bed or a change from familiar surroundings to a hospital ward. Incontinence usually disappears with the cure of the acute illness but in about 10 per cent of cases the condition persists.

### Causes of persistent urinary incontinence

**Neurological disease.** Bladder function is under the control of the autonomic nervous system (Fig. 14.1). As the bladder dilates with urine, information is transmitted to the spinal cord by afferent fibres. This produces direct stimulation of efferent fibres and consequent smooth-muscle contraction and bladder emptying. The process can be enhanced or inhibited by fibres linking the local reflex with voluntary centres in the cerebral cortex. Damage to any part of this system can result in incontinence.

(a) *Cerebral cortex.* Damage at this level reduces the suppressant effect of the brain on the local spinal cord reflex. Pressure within the bladder is increased, causing the bladder to empty more frequently. The main causes of cortical damage in the elderly are brain failure and cerebrovascular damage (Chapter 9).

(b) *Spinal cord.* Partial destruction of fibres in the spinal cord causes a change in bladder function similar to that due to cortical damage. Complete interruption of the fibres in the spinal cord causes a loss of voluntary control over bladder emptying, and in this situation the bladder has a high pressure and empties spontaneously at frequent intervals. Complete

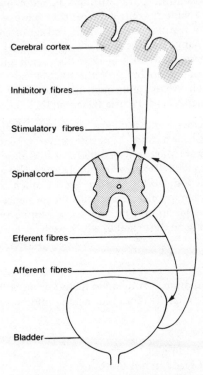

Figure 14.1   CNS pathways controlling
bladder function

destruction of the spinal cord pathways due to trauma or disseminated sclerosis is relatively uncommon in old people, but patchy damage due to a poor blood supply or pressure from a prolapsed disc or early tumour is much more common.

(c) *Afferent fibres.* Destruction of afferent fibres results in a breakdown of the local bladder reflex arc. Smooth-muscle fibres do not then contract in response to bladder dilation, and the bladder fills until it can fill no longer. Any further urine simply leaks out of the bladder, and the patient experiences a continuous dribbling incontinence. The most common cause of this condition are diabetes and Parkinson's disease (Chapter 13).

**Local causes.** Local factors are important, often remediable, causes of incontinence. The most common is faecal impaction, where pressure of a loaded rectum on the urethra and bladder interferes with the local reflex and either acute retention or frank urinary incontinence may result. Old women are often unable to control micturition because of a weakened or damaged pelvic floor, and in this situation, leakage often follows laughing or coughing or a change in posture (stress incontinence). Males may suffer from prostatic enlargement with bladder distension and overflow incontinence. In women hypertrophy of the bladder neck causes a similar outflow obstruction. An acute urinary infection may cause incontinence by inducing frequency and dysuria (Chapter 13: *urinary infection*).

**Environmental factors.** Incontinence is often accentuated by the interaction between ill-health and a hostile environment. Immobility is extremely important. Many old people have difficulty in getting to the lavatory quickly enough. This is particularly important after a cerebrovascular accident where disability is often accompanied by bladder hyperactivity. Diuretic therapy also accentuates incontinence. The design and layout of accommodation and the amount of supporting care available have a direct bearing on the extent to which such factors create problems.

### Investigation

**History and examination.** A detailed history from both the patient and his relatives is essential. This should include information about:

*Voiding*
(a) Onset
(b) Relief after voiding
(c) Sensation of bladder and urethra
(d) Initiation of micturition
(e) Enuresis
(f) Use of catheter or urinal

*Type of incontinence*
(a) Precipitant micturition
(b) Psychological
(c) Stress
(d) Overflow
(e) Reflex
(f) Incontinence of non-resistance, i.e. dribbling

*Bowel history*
(a) Frequency
(b) Desire to defaecate

(c) Differentiation of gas from faeces
(d) Anal sensation
(e) Interruption (in the presence of diarrhoea)

Physical examination, especially that of the central nervous system, should be thorough. Particular attention should be paid to the size of the bladder and to whether or not the prostate is enlarged or the rectum

| INCONTINENCE CHART | | | | | | | | |
|---|---|---|---|---|---|---|---|---|
| Surname: SMITH | | | First Names: JOHN | | | Unit No:  130475 | | |
| | | | | | | Ward      F Ward | | |
| Date:      1.1.86 | | | 2.1.86 | | 3.1.86 | | 4.1.86 | |
| Time | Commode ·or bed pan given by | U.F. or dry | Commode or bed pan given by | U.F. or dry | Commode or bed pan given by | U.F. or dry | Commode or bed pan given by | U.F. or dry |
| A.M. 0800 | | | | D | | | | |
| 1000 | | U | | | | U | | U |
| P.M. 1200 | | U | | U | | | | U |
| 1400 | | D | | D | | D | | |
| 1600 | | | | D | | D | | |
| 1800 | | D | | D | | D | | |
| 2000 | | | | D | | | | D |
| 2200 | | | | | | | | |
| 2400 | | | | | | | | |
| A.M. 0200 | | | | | | | | |
| 0400 | | | | | | D | | |

Figure 14.2    Incontinence chart

contains faeces. In women, vaginal examination plays an important part in the assessment. Laboratory tests should include urinalysis and culture of the urine (Chapter 13).

**Incontinence Pattern** (Case 2). An incontinence chart (Fig. 14.2) should be kept, on which any episodes of urinary or faecal incontinence should be recorded, thus providing information on their severity and timing. The chart should also contain details of the times when patients either visited the lavatory or were given a bedpan or bottle and, if possible, the amount of urine they passed. This will allow an accurate assessment of the severity of any urinary frequency as well as bladder capacity.

**Cystometrography** (Cases 2, 3). Measurement of pressure within the bladder and urethra may also be of great value. Figure 14.3 illustrates a simple technique whereby this can be done. The patient is asked to micturate, after which a catheter is introduced and any urine remaining in the bladder is drained and measured. The end of the catheter is then linked by a 'Y' connection to a reservoir of lukewarm saline and to a free tube marked in centimetres of water; 25 ml of saline is introduced to the blad-

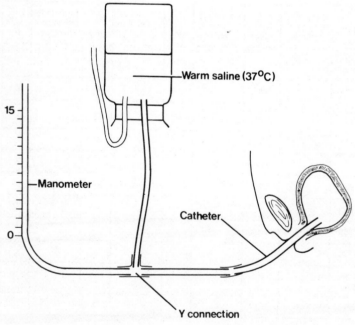

Figure 14.3  Cystometrography

der and a pressure recording made. The process is repeated, adding a further 25 ml each time until the patient expresses a desire to void urine. Bladder sensation can be assessed by introducing chilled saline and ask-

Table 14.1 Cystometrography Patterns in Normal and Neurogenic Bladders

|  | Normal bladder | Uninhibited bladder | Atonic bladder |
| --- | --- | --- | --- |
| Resting bladder pressure | <10 cm $H_2O$ | >10 cm $H_2O$ | <10 cm $H_2O$ |
| Desire to void urine | 350 ml | <250 ml | Absent |
| Bladder capacity | <600 ml | 600 ml | >800 ml |
| Response to stretch | Nil | Rise in pressure | Nil |

ing the patient to differentiate it from warm fluid. Table 14.1 details the recordings to be found in different types of bladder.

In the normal bladder there is a low resting pressure which remains low until the patient experiences a desire to void urine. Increased bladder activity is associated with a high resting pressure which rises with each increase in volume, and the patient experiences a desire to micturate at a reduced volume. The capacity of patients with atonic bladders is increased, there is no sensation, and no change in pressure as volume increases.

The simple technique described above has severe limitations in that it does not provide a continuous record of bladder volume and pressure, and does not take into account changes in the intra-abdominal pressure unrelated to bladder tone. For these reasons, many geriatric units now make use of electronic transducers and recorders. With these it is possible to measure intravesical and intrarectal pressures concurrently, and use a simple subtraction technique to estimate the bladder tone.

It is also possible to take serial measurements of pressure as the catheter is withdrawn from the bladder and thus assess transurethral pressure. The transurethral pressure profile may be useful in aiding diagnosis and assessing the efficacy of treatment.

**Radiology** (Case 2). An intravenous pyelogram provides information on any renal abnormality. At the completion of this test detailed information on bladder function can be obtained by X-raying the organ before and after micturition. The normal bladder has a smooth outline and a horizontal base. In hyperactivity, there are often multiple diverticula and trabeculae, the base is funnelled and there usually is some residual urine after micturition. Prostatic enlargement is also associated with trabeculae and diverticula, with the enlarged gland in evidence as an indentation at the base of the bladder, after micturition a large quantity of contrast medium remains in the bladder. Radiology is also useful in identifying bladder calculi and tumours.

**Cytoscopy.** Examination of the state of the bladder by direct vision can sometimes be useful when doubt exists as to the exact cause of the incontinence. Close co-operation beween genito-urinary surgical teams and geriatric medical teams is essential if the right decisions are to be made for many incontinent patients.

## Treatment

**Environmental changes** (Case 2; Chapter 5). The treatment if incontinence varies with the aetiology. Where mobility is a problem, care must be taken to ensure that the patient has ready access to the lavatory. This may involve the provision of a commode at home. Whenever possible, however, attempts should be made to adapt the lavatory to the patient's needs. If the lavatory is inaccessible, consideration should be given to moving to more suitable housing. Admission to an institution should be preceded by a visit to ensure that all parts of the building likely to be used by the patient are within easy reach of a lavatory.

**Diuretic therapy** (Case 2). Diuretic therapy should, wherever feasible, be avoided in incontinent patients, but if it cannot considerable care should be exercised in the selection. The diuretic used should be governed by the pattern of incontinence: if incontinence occurs at night a short-acting diuretic is best, and a long-acting diuretic is preferable in the disabled patient who has difficulty in getting to the lavatory. Selection of a suitable agent can be very difficult, because the normal strength and duration of action for a diuretic is often affected by age-related changes in its absorption, metabolism and excretion (Chapter 5). Close surveillance is of more value than reliance on information from pharmacological textbooks.

**Bowel function.** The relief of faecal impaction is essential in the control of urinary incontinence and can often be achieved by the administration of an enema. Manual evacuation may sometimes be necessary.

**Toilet training** (Case 3). Training plays an important part in the management of an incontinent patient, and is particularly relevant in situations where bladder capacity is limited by hyperactivity or sphincter weakness. Such patients should be encouraged to visit the lavatory once every two hours. In certain instances, indeed, it may be necessary to wake the patient during the course of the night, but the inconvenience of being wakened before incontinence occurs is less than the distress of waking in a bed soaked with urine.

Bedpans should be avoided. Micturition or defaecation into them is physiologically and psychologically difficult. Their use also takes the responsibility for bowel and bladder control away from the patient, and causes increased dependence on nursing staff. The same objection applies to the use of urinals.

Commodes have a limited value in the management of severely disabled people at home. In most other situations they should be avoided, for they encourage the patient to consider himself a permanent invalid and act as a disincentive to achieving mobility and independence.

**Drugs** (Case 3). It would seem likely that cholinergic and anti-cholinergic drugs would alter bladder function by increasing or decreasing tone, but their success in the control of incontinence has been limited. Cholinergic agents (eg. bethanechol) certainly increase bladder tonus but do not restore sensitivity. The anti-cholinergics (propantheline, imipramine) may be helpful in reducing the severity and frequency of incontinence in the hyperactive bladder, but are rarely effective if used in isolation; they are best employed as an adjunct to the training methods already described. Other drugs such as quinestradol (Pentovis) may help to normalise bladder epithelium, thereby perhaps increasing sensitivity, while laxatives and faecal softeners have an important role in preventing constipation and faecal impaction.

**Surgery** (Case 6). Prostatectomy by a transurethral resection should be considered whenever incontinence is due to prostatic enlargement. The age of the patient is no barrier to this type of surgery. The operation should always be preceded by adequate investigation of bladder function. If the patient with an enlarged prostrate also has a hypertonic bladder due to coincidental neurological disease, prostatectomy will accentuate rather than alleviate the urinary incontinence.

Surgery should be considered in women where stress incontinence is due to a lax pelvic floor and when retention with overflow occurs as a result of bladder neck obstruction, but as with prostatectomy care should be taken beforehand to ensure that the local lesion is the true cause of the incontinence. A ring pessary may be inserted in cases of stress incontinence when surgery is impracticable.

**Physiotherapy.** Pelvic floor exercises may be of value in helping some women with stress incontinence to control their bladder outlet. Patients however need to co-operate with the physiotherapist who in turn needs to have experience of these exercises.

**Faradic stimulation.** Various electrical devices have been used to increase tonus in muscles of the pelvic floor by Faradic stimulation. These are inserted in either the rectum or the vagina and connected to a battery. They are worth a trial in stress or post-prostatectomy incontinence but their effectiveness is often disappointing.

**Urinals.** Where incontinence cannot be controlled, steps should be taken to minimise the incontinence and the embarrassment it causes. Males can often be fitted with a urinal attached to a leg bag. Where nocturnal incontinence is a problem, an apparatus with a non-return valve should be fitted. Mental capacity and manual dexterity are of major importance to a patient adapting to such a device, and a considerable amount of training by both nurse and occupational therapist may be necessary before the individual becomes self-sufficient.

**Incontinence pads.** No practical urinal has yet been developed for the incontinent female, and resort has to be had to water-absorbent materials. The simplest form of this is the incontinence pad and which comprises a sheet of water-absorbent paper and waterproof backing. Although this pad only absorbs a very limited quantity of urine it can be of considerable value in reducing the amount of laundering necessary for bedfast patients with relatively mild incontinence.

Considerable research has been expended on developing materials capable of absorbing large quantities of urine. A polygel material has been produced recently in the form of a pad which is worn in a marsupial pouch attached to pants (Kanga pants). It is extremely effective in elderly women with mild to moderate degrees of stress incontinence.

**Catheterisation.** Where all else fails, catheterisation should be considered. This may be the only way of getting a patient back home, or of healing macerated skin. It is doubtful whether this measure should ever be used merely to cut down laundry expenses or reduce the nursing workload.

Catheterisation is usually followed by urinary infection, and persistent infection will ultimately cause chronic renal failure. Consideration should be given to the life expectancy of the patient; where this is low, the long-term consequences of catherisation can be ignored.

Where catheterisation is employed, infection is best minimised by using a meticulous aseptic technique, by changing the catheter regularly and by using Silastic rather than rubber catheters. Urine should be allowed to drain freely into a non-returnable leg bag, or into a bag attached around the waist (Shepherd's sporran). Intermittent catheter drainage, by causing bladder stasis, is invariably followed by infection. It should be avoided where catheterisation is permanent but may be useful when it is ultimately intended to withdraw the catheter and restore continence. Four-hourly emptying prevents the bladder from becoming small and hypertonic. Bladder washouts are of little value in preventing infection and are best avoided as a routine measure.

Table 14.2   Causes of Faecal Incontinence

Faecal impaction
Diarrhoea due to: dietary indiscretion
       bacterial or viral infection
       purgative abuse
       diverticular disease
       cancer
Leakage of liquid paraffin
Damage to pelvic floor with: lax anal sphincter
           rectal prolapse
Loss of colonic inhibition due to: dementia
            cord damage

## Faecal incontinence

Faecal incontinence is much less common than loss of bladder control.
Table 14.2 lists causes in the elderly, the most important of these being
faecal impaction.

## Faecal impaction (Cases 1, 3, 5)

Increasing age is associated with slowing in the transit of food through
the gastro-intestinal tract. The exact cause for this is unclear, and it is
doubtful whether there are any age-related changes in colonic mobility.
Possible factors include a reduction in dietary roughage and a decrease in
physical exercise. The main effect of delayed transit is the accumulation of
hard dehydrated faeces in the rectum and sigmoid colon.

Faecal impaction is further accentuated in patients neglecting a call to
stool, as happens in disabled patients who experience difficulty in getting
to a lavatory. Those who are bedfast have the problem of using a bedpan,
when effective defaecation is dependent on a human assuming the
crouching position. Finally, sheer physical weakness may make faecal
evacuation difficult.

Faecal incontinence due to impaction presents as the leakage of liquid
faeces from the anus, as fluid material in the more proximal part of the
colon bypasses the concretions lower down. The diagnosis is made by
identifying hard faeces in the rectum or lower part of the colon. In addition to digital examination of the rectum, a plain abdominal X-ray can be
helpful in making the diagnosis.

**Treatment.**   The condition can usually be treated by using an enema.
Soap and water enemas should never be used, for they may cause a
disastrous dehydration and haemoconcentration; small hypertonic phosphate enemas are equally effective and are virtually free from side effects.

An example is Fletcher's Phosphate Enema (sodium acid phosphate 12.8 g, sodium phosphate 10.24 g dissolved in 128 ml water). Very occasionally, manual evacuation of faeces may be a necessary preliminary to the administration of an enema.

Once the colon has been emptied of faeces, regularity must be maintained. Traditionally, this task is often left to nursing staff, and while it is appropriate for nurses to continue to supervise bowel function, accurate records must be kept and bowel control reviewed regularly on ward rounds, case conferences or home visits, so that appropriate régimes may be prescribed by doctors.

A wide range of laxatives is available but relatively few are of value in old age.

(a) *Bran.* Colonic roughage can be increased by encouraging the consumption of fruit, prunes and fibrous cereals. Bran is an extremely effective agent (Chapter 12).

(b) *Lactulose.* Faecal bulk can also be increased by using lactulose. Fermentation of this synthetic disaccharide in the colon produces frequent soft stools. It also produces gas which often gives rise to flatulence, and abdominal discomfort. The dose should be related to the response (Chapter 5).

(c) *Stool softeners and lubricants.* Old people experience difficulty in passing hard faeces, and stool-softening agents can be of value in this situation. Liquid paraffin was used for many years, but if aspirated it can cause pneumonia and taken in excess or incorrectly it causes anal leakage. It has no place in present day treatment.

Dioctyl sodium sulphosuccinate is an effective softening agent with few proven side effects. Concern has been expressed on its possible long-term effects on gastro-intestinal absorption, but these are of theoretical rather than practical significance. Dosage is 200 mg three times a day initially, reducing to 200 mg on alternate days.

Saline purgatives are of considerable pharmacological interest, but have little place in modern clinical practice.

(d) *Irritant laxatives.* Drugs with a local irritant effect on the colon seem to be reasonably effective as laxatives. Standardised senna in a dose of one or two tablets daily is a suitable preparation, although some patients prefer equivalent doses of senna in granules or a syrup. Bisacodyl in a dose of one to two tablets is a useful alternative. More powerful irritants such as castor oil are of historical interest; they have no place in present-day therapy.

Patients with bowel problems should receive advice on preventing a recurrence of impaction. They should visit the lavatory once a day and attempt to pass faeces whether or not they feel the call. In ensuring that the patient complies with this, arrangements should be made for him to have easy access to the lavatory. This may involve putting up rails, building an inside lavatory, supplying a commode or moving him to more suitable accomodation.

Considerable stress should be laid on the dangers of laxative overdosage. Examples of potassium depletion or defective gut innervation (melanosis coli) resulting from this habit are by no means rare in geriatric wards, and emphasis on the normality of passing a motion less frequently than once a day in old age may reduce the incidence of the problem. Finally, a general improvement in health and mobility go a long way to preventing a recurrence of faecal impaction, for the condition is predominantly a disorder of the sick and the chairbound.

**Diarrhoea.** Old people may become incontinent of faeces as a result of diarrhoea. Investigation and appropriate treatment of the cause invariably controls the situation. This may appear self-evident, but some old people are labelled 'senile' or 'demented' simply because faeces are found on their bed clothes – yet another example of the dangers of attributing symptoms of old age to ageing. Symptomatic treatment with antidiarrhoeal drugs may be indicated to alleviate the patient's distress while investigation is taking place.

**Mental impairment.** A few patients with mental impairment may simply defaecate in inappropriate situations. This only occurs where organic brain disease has reached an advanced stage, and even here attempts should always be made to exclude remediable causes for the incontinence. Where none can be found, the problem can sometimes be reduced by producing constipation with a standard mixture of kaolin and morphine in a dose of 15 ml daily, inducing passive bowel evacuation by the weekly administration of a saline enema.

## Further reading

Avery Jones F & Godding E W (1973) *Management of Constipation*. Oxford: Blackwell Scientific Publications

Brocklehurst J C (1984) *Urology in the Elderly*. Edinburgh: Churchill Livingstone

Mandelstram D (1980) *Incontinence and its Management*. London: Croom Helm

Willington F L (1976) *Incontinence in the Elderly*. London: Academic Press

# CHAPTER 15

# Terminal Care

The death rate in most geriatric units is about 30 per cent, and as the proportion of the very old in the population increases this figure is likely to rise. It would seem important, therefore, that doctors, nurses and social workers looking after the elderly should study the problems of pain, death and bereavement.

## The management of the dying

The treatment of the dying patient raises many ethical issues, the individual's approach to these being governed by his cultural background and general attitude to life. Dogmatic pronouncements are inappropriate to this aspect of medical and nursing care, but despite this, considerable training, experience, skill and judgement is involved in the management of terminal illness and the handling of bereaved relatives. An increasing proportion of doctors, nurses and social workers have developed an interest in this difficult field, and their writings have provided us with many useful and practical guidelines.

**To treat or not to treat?** (Case 4).   A doctor is sometimes faced with the question of whether or not he should treat a particular illness at all, for by treatment he may not prolong life, but merely produce a more lingering death. The difficulty is that decisions often have to be taken with inadequate information. The noisy, confused elderly patient may have been severely demented for several years; his condition, on the other hand, may be entirely related to the recent onset of an acute medical condition. It is important that as much information as possible should be obtained about his past history from relatives, neighbours, general practitioners, district nurses, health visitors, social workers and home helps before treatment is begun.

The choice is rarely between treatment and no treatment. Even where the decision is taken not to prevent death, active measures must be taken to prevent suffering. Thus it may be necessary to treat to relieve breathlessness in terminal pneumonia, to control obstruction of the vena cava in lung cancer or to relieve the pain of bony secondaries.

**What to tell the patient** (Case 4).   A great deal of attention has been given to the question of whether or not a patient should be told that he is dying. An important consideration is the nature of the illness. If the disorder is associated with gross intellectual impairment, discussion with the patient is futile. Again, if a rapid decline is associated with a degenerative condition such as coronary artery disease, accurate prediction of the time and nature of death is impossible. Even if the patient has cancer, prognostication can be fraught with difficulty, for progression of a tumour may be extremely slow in old age. Many people with cancer of the breast or prostate live for years after the diagnosis is made, and may often die from causes completely unrelated to their cancer.

Despite these exceptions, there remains a small group of alert patients in whom the outcome is clear. The least exacting line of approach is for the relatives and supporting staff to maintain a facade of false optimism, but this is rarely effective and they are ultimately forced into inventing a whole web of fabrication. Once the patient detects the deception he will lose faith in all concerned, and his behaviour alters; he may simply give up asking questions. More usually, to avoid embarrassment he plays everyone else's game pretending that he believes that he has a favourable prognosis. This may place a barrier between the patient and his attendants and relatives and he may have to face the ultimate crisis alone and unsupported.

Unvarnished frankness may also lead to considerable distress. Pronouncement of a death sentence is often followed by a period of unbelief and denial. When the truth becomes apparent the patient may struggle against the inevitable by going from doctor to doctor, by attempting to bargain for his life with a deity, or by altering life-long habits to which he may relate his illness. When this fails, he may seek an alternative target for his predicament which, all too often, emerges as a close relative; nursing and medical staff may also be involved. Such people may seek escape by complete withdrawal and depression.

Supporting staff can do much to avoid this sequence of events by understanding the patient, his family and his dilemma. An appropriate starting point may be a discussion of the prognosis with a close relative, who can provide information on the patient's personality and his probable reaction to the terminal illness. He can then be approached and be given an explanation as to the general nature of this illness. Dependent upon his reaction, it may be possible to go on to discuss the prognosis with him. Sometimes he will not want to know and will accept explanations even though suspecting the worst. Direct lies should always be avoided. Hope for a normal, comfortable life should never be destroyed.

The length of the discussion varies. In a few instances it may be possible to make a complete exposition within a few sentences. More often, the details should emerge over a period of several days or weeks. It is important that the information a patient gleans from different members of the staff should not contain major discrepancies. Detailed notes of all important conversations are absolutely essential to achieve this; these should be kept in case records to which all members of the staff have access and to which they should contribute. A separate sheet of a distinguishing colour may prove a useful addition to the notes. All staff can then write a summary of their communication with relatives and patient on this.

**Relief of symptoms** (Case 4).    Sympathetic discussion is of little avail if the patient remains uncomfortable and distressed. People looking after dying patients should be skilled in the use of analgesic and psychotropic drugs, their objective being to achieve the maximum of relief from pain with a minimum of clouding of consciousness.

Relatively mild analgesics can often be used if these are given in regular doses; they are less effective if given only when pain recurs, and in this situation the patient comes to dread the return of pain. Anxiety, coupled with a psychological adaptation to the drug, results in his requiring ever larger doses and the doctor is eventually confronted with the choice of either making him unconscious or leaving him in pain. Regular dosage at adequate levels will minimise both anxiety and drug tolerance.

Table 15.1 lists some of the drugs of value in the relief of pain. In addition to these, sustained release morphine (MST Continus) tablets may be useful in reducing the number of doses required and, in particular, in allowing the patient to sleep through the night without being wakened for a repeat dose of morphine. It should be remembered that aspirin is often very effective in relieving bone pain associated with bony secondaries. Steroids may also be helpful in producing euphoria or a sense of well-being as well as reducing hypercalcaemia associated with bone secondaries associated with carcinoma of the breast. The fact that an agent is narcotic should not be a barrier to its administration. Even heroin (diamorphine) given for several months, does not produce addiction in terminal illness so long as doses are given regularly and kept at the minimum necessary for effective pain relief.

Pain is often associated with anxiety. Sympathy and explanation will help to relieve this, and tranquillisers may occasionally be used (Table 15.2 lists some suitable agents). Barbiturates are best avoided, for they

Table 15.1   Analgesics

| Drug | Analgesic effect | Anxiolytic effect | Dose | Route | Side effects |
|---|---|---|---|---|---|
| Aspirin | + | — | 600 mg | Oral | — |
| Paracetamol | + | — | 0.5–1 gm | Oral | — |
| Codeine | + | — | 30 mg | Oral | Constipation |
| Dihydrocodeine | ++ | — | 30–60 mg | Oral | Constipation |
| Pentazocine | + | — | 30 mg | IM | — |
| Pentazocine | ++ | — | 25–100 mg | Oral | — |
| Methadone linctus | ++ | — | 5–10 mg | Oral | — |
| Pethidine | ++ | — | 50–100 mg | IM | — |
| Morphine | +++ | +++ | 8–20 mg | SC | Vomiting, constipation |
| Diamorphine | +++ | +++ | 5–10 mg | IM | — |
| Morphine mixture* | +++ | +++ | 15–25 ml | Oral | — |

* 15 ml contains 15 mg morphine and 15 ml chloroform water
Note: Only side effects likely to be of importance in terminal illness are recorded

Table 15.2   Oral Tranquillisers

| Drug | Daily dosage |
|------|-------------|
| Chlorpromazine | 25–50 mg |
| Thioridazine | 10–50 mg |
| Promazine | 50 mg |
| Diazepam | 2–15 mg |
| Chlordiazepoxide | 5–40 mg |

produce sedation and there is also good evidence that far from relieving pain they tend to accentuate it.

Attention should also be directed to other distressing symptoms associated with terminal illness. Breathlessness should be dealt with by treating the cause. If, following this, the condition persists or is associated with a painful cough, suppression of respiration with a narcotic preparation such as methodone linctus should be considered. Here, a balance between relieving distress and accelerating death may have to be struck.

Vomiting is a distressing feature of many terminal illnesses, and Table 15.3 lists some useful anti-emetic agents. Hyoscine, although an antimetic, causes restlessness and confusion in old people and should not be used. If the symptom is due to gastro-intestinal obstruction palliative surgery should always be considered, the discomfort of an operation having to be balanced against the distress of persistent vomiting and starvation. Metabolic causes such as elevation of the blood calcium must also be remembered.

Terminal illness is often associated with gross wasting due to a combination of increased protein breakdown and a poor nutrient intake. It is usually followed by the onset of pressure sores. Anabolic drugs, such as the oral agent stanozolol, merit consideration; they not only reduce weight loss, but often have a mild euphoriant effect. Tissue breakdown can be further delayed by the administration of ascorbic acid. In addition to these measures, good general nursing care is essential in the prevention of pressure sores (Chapter 5).

Table 15.3   Oral Anti-emetics

| Drug | Sedative effect | Dose |
|------|-----------------|------|
| Chlorpromazine | + | 25–50 mg |
| Promazine | + | 50–100 mg |
| Cyclizine | ++ | 25–50 mg |
| Metoclopramide | – | 5–10 mg |
| Domperidone | – | 10–30 mg |

Note: None of these drugs has side effects that are likely to be of importance in terminal illness.

## Bereavement

Concern should also be directed at the relatives of the dying patient. This is particularly important where a relative is elderly, and even more important where she is physically or mentally frail. Bereavement is usually associated with a sense of loss and of loneliness which may go on to produce a true depression. Equally distressing is the sense of guilt which often accompanies bereavement, especially common where the illness has been prolonged and the relative experiences relief at the time of death, or where hospital admission immediately preceded death. The stress of bereavement may also cause very real physical illness, and there is even an increased death rate in close relatives during the first year of bereavement.

These hazards can be reduced by closely following up a relative for some time after the death of a patient. Treatment usually consists of providing sympathy and giving advice about readjusting to changed circumstances. Tranquillisers may be useful in the earlier stages of bereavement but their administration should be judicious; they should be given to help the subject to work through the normal process of mourning. Grief is a healthy reaction and should be encouraged. Indeed, there may be advantages in sharing this with the dying relative before death. Total suppression of grief may result in its effects being even more distressing later on. If after several months the subject remains severely distressed the possibility of depression should be considered; this often exhibits a gratifying response to anti-depressant drugs.

## Malignancy

The incidence of many malignant conditions rises with increasing age. Some, such as lung cancer, reach a peak incidence in late middle age and show a decreasing frequency in extreme old age.

Malignancy in the elderly differs from that in the rest of the population in several important respects.

1 tumours often grow more slowly in old age;
2 because of the limited life expectancy of old people, many with cancer die from causes unrelated to the cancer; and
3 reduced pain sensation and a diminished inflammatory response may allow a tumour to reach a later stage in its development and to spread to other areas before it causes symptoms and is diagnosed.

**Breast cancer.** Breast cancer often progresses very slowly in old age. Surgery is rarely indicated since most cases show a satisfactory response to the anti-oestrogen agent, tamoxifen, given in a dose of 10 mg twice daily.

Bony secondaries are a common cause of distress in elderly women and may give rise to hypercalcaemia (*see above: relief of symptoms*). The cancer may present as a fractured shaft or neck of femur which may require surgical treatment with fixation or irradiation. Metastases are often hormone dependent, and often respond to tamoxifen.

**Lung cancer.**   This condition often presents in the elderly in a variety of bizarre and unexpected ways. Details of its diagnosis and management are discussed in Chapter 11.

**Cancer of the prostate.**   This condition bears a very close relationship to ageing. Post-mortem studies have identified latent changes in 95 per cent of men over the age of 90 years. Fortunately, it usually remains localised and frequently gives rise to no symptoms at all. Where the condition is localised and symptoms are present local surgery may be indicated.

Symptoms such as bone pain, lethargy, malaise and pallor due to anaemia, are more frequently related to bony secondaries than to bladder obstruction. The growth rate of secondaries may be extremely slow in old age; they also show a high degree of hormone dependency, and symptoms respond well when the patient is given small doses of stilboestrol. Thus the prognosis for the condition is good, and patients survive with minimal symptoms for many years.

**Multiple myeloma.**   Multiple myeloma is a proliferative disease involving marrow plasma cells, and should always be considered when a patient has a high ESR; this is usually in excess of 100 mm/1st hour, but lower values may sometimes be recorded. Radiology can be misleading in old age. Fractures or collapsed vertebrae are common, but these are often accompanied by generalised bone rarefaction which disguises the focal areas of rarefaction characteristic of the disease. A high index of suspicion is necessary in this situation. The diagnosis can usually be confirmed by looking for abnormal protein bands in the plasma and by identifying the abnormal plasma cells in a marrow aspiration. Patients often show a good temporary response to chemotherapy.

**Chronic lymphatic leukaemia.**   The condition may exist without symptoms, but the first evidence of it is usually the identification of a very high lymphocyte count in a sample of blood taken for routine haematological investigation. A diagnosis can usually be established by marrow aspiration or by lymph node biopsy. The condition tends to progress very slowly and treatment is hardly ever necessary in old age. However, patients with white cell counts of over 20,000/mm³ should be followed up carefully and treatment considered if recurrent infections, particularly respiratory infection, occur.

## Further reading

Copperman H (1984) *Dying at Home*. Chichester: Wiley
Hinton J (1967) *Dying*. Harmondsworth: Penguin (Pelican) Books
Murray Parkes C (1985) Terminal care: home, hospital or hospice? *Lancet*, **1**, 155–157
Saunders C (1984) *The Management of Terminal Illness*. London: Edward Arnold
Wilkes E (1980) *Terminal Care*. Report of the Working Group, Standing Medical Advisory Committee. DHSS: London

# Index